Readers' Praise

"Exceptional!!! A must read for all those who seek to enhance their health and prevent disease."

—Dr. Stephen Nenninger
New York, New York

"Practical, and in an easy-to-understand manner, Dr. Mark Stengler provides direction and expert advice on the application of natural methods of healing in relieving common health problems."

—Dr. Tori Hudson
Professor, National College of Naturopathic Medicine
Portland, Oregon

"Incredible—it works! I've suffered the aggravation and discomfort of irritable bowel syndrome for many years. I've spent countless hours travelling to other communities to see specialists, been tested, poked and prodded, and tried many prescriptions to no avail. I was ready to try anything to ease my pain and discomfort when I heard Dr. Stengler on a local radio show. After four days on the naturopathic routine that Dr. Stengler prescribed, I noticed an amazing improvement in my condition and today, I feel better than I've felt in five years! Thank you Dr. Stengler!"

—Miss Janice Flemming
Medicine Hat, Alberta

The Natural Physician

Your Health Guide for Common Ailments

Mark Stengler, ND

Foreword by Lendon H. Smith, MD

The
Natural
Physician

Your Health Guide
for Common Ailments

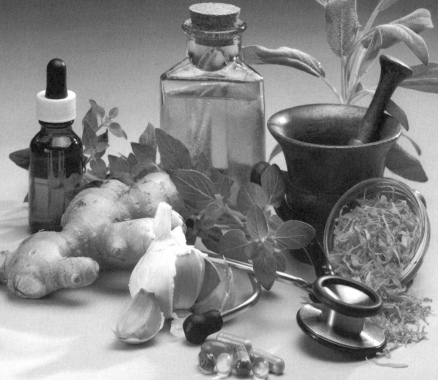

Mark Stengler, ND
Foreword by Lendon H. Smith, MD

alive
books

The information in this book is intended to be used as an educational resource only. It is not to be used as a replacement for professional medical evaluation and treatment. Consult with your physician before following any therapy in this book. The majority of the recommended dosages in this manual are written for adults. Conditions unique to infants such as colic include the appropriate recommended dosages. Women who are pregnant, expecting pregnancy or nursing should only follow the advice of their medical professional.

Published by
Alive Books
PO Box 80055
Burnaby, BC Canada V5H 3X1

Designer: Kerstin Barth
Cover Photo: Siegfried Gursche
Back Cover Photo: Sandy Wright

Printing, first edition: October 1997
"The Natural Physician" is a registered trademark of Dr. Mark Stengler.
All rights reserved.

Canadian Cataloguing in Publication Data

Stengler, Mark
 The natural physician

Includes bibliographical references and index.
ISBN 0-920470-46-7

1. Naturopathy–Popular works. 2. Alternative medicine
Popular works. I. Title.
RZ440.S73 1997   615.5'35   C97-910538-2

Printed and bound in Canada

Acknowledgements

My path as a physician began when I was introduced to a naturopathic doctor through **Lorna** and **Dave Bridarolli**. My thanks to them.

I would like to acknowledge all the doctors and professors who nurtured my medical training. Many brilliant naturopathic physicians, and other health care practitioners I have worked with, often go without recognition as they improve the quality of life for humankind.

A grateful thanks to my friends and colleagues **Dr. Roseanne** and **Steve Nenninger** for their support. To **Dr. Marcus Laux** for his leadership in the field of natural medicine.

To **Donald Cranston**, **Pages Publishing**, and **Siegfried Gursche** and **Katherine Zia** of **Alive Books** for their support.

A special thanks to my brilliant editor **Catherine Southwood** for her expertise and patience.

My special appreciation to the **Ragusa** and **Hart families**. A special thanks to all my friends; my parents **Mary** and **Art Stengler**; to my family—**Barb, Steve, Ryan, Nicholas, Kris, Darcy, Tyler, Jordan, Brooklyn, Wade, Kevin** and **Logan**; grandparents **Nick** and **Eleanor Stengler** and **Margaret Bechal**.

To my beautiful wife **Angela** for her incredible support and love. You are very patient and kind. Your encouragement is much appreciated.

Table of Contents

Foreword by Lendon H. Smith, MD . . . . *xii*
Preface by Tori Hudson, ND . . . . *xiii*
Introduction 1
The Naturopathic Physician 3
Principles of Naturopathic Medicine 7

Using This Guide 9
Acne 9
Alzheimer's 11
Anemia 13
Angina 14
Anxiety 16
Arthritis (Osteoarthritis) 18
Asthma 20
Atherosclerosis 22
Athlete's Foot 24
Athletic Performance Enhancement 25
Bites and Stings 28
Black Eye 29
Boils 30
Bronchitis 31
Bruises 32
Burns 33
Bursitis 34
Cancer 36
Canker Sores 39
Carpal Tunnel Syndrome 40
Cataracts 42
Cervical Dysplasia 43
Cold 45
Cold Sores 47
Colic 48
Constipation 50

Cough 51
Cuts 53
Dandruff 53
Depression 55
Diabetes 57
Diarrhea 59
Ear Infections 60
Fatigue 62
Fever 64
Fibrocystic Breast Disease 65
Food Allergies and Sensitivities 67
Fractures 68
Gallstones 70
Gout 71
Gum Disease (Gingivitis) 73
Headache 74
Heartburn 76
Heart Disease 77
Hemorrhoids 79
High Blood Pressure (Hypertension) 81
HIV (AIDS) 83
Hyperactivity (ADHD) 85
Hypothyroid 86
Impotence 88
Indigestion 90
Insomnia 91
Irritable Bowel Syndrome (IBS) 93
Jet Lag 95
Kidney Stones 96
Lupus 98
Menopause 99
Menstrual Cramps 101
Multiple Sclerosis 103
Muscle Cramps 105
Nausea 107
Osteoporosis 108

Pink Eye (Conjunctivitis) 110
PMS (Premenstrual Syndrome) 112
Prostate Enlargement 113
Psoriasis 115
Rash 116
Sinusitis 118
Sore Throat 119
Sprains and Strains 121
Stress 123
TMJ Syndrome 124
Ulcers 126
Urinary Tract Infection 128
Varicose Veins 130
Warts 131
Weight Loss 133
Yeast Infection (Vaginitis) 136

Appendix A Natural Physician Hydrotherapy Guide 139
Appendix B Natural Physician Homeopathy Guide 144
Appendix C Natural Physician Herbal Medicine Guide 154
Appendix D Natural Physician Healthy Diet Guidelines ...166
Appendix E Food Allergies and Sensitivities
Elimination and Reintroduction Diet 170
Appendix F Natural Physician Vitamin and Mineral Guide .173
Appendix G Natural Physician Guide to Choosing Quality
Supplements 195

Glossary 198
Resources 206
References 207
Index 208
About the Author 217
Other Titles by Alive 218

Foreword

Conventional medical doctors have noted that their patients are asking embarrassing questions like: Is there a natural method for treating my symptoms? Why do I get sick on prescription drugs? Why don't they work well? Why are they so expensive? This guide to the use of natural remedies has come along at exactly the right time to help patients and even to allow medical doctors to feel more comfortable when a patient asks for alternative treatments.

There are choices in health care. By using this book and following the advice of Dr. Stengler, a conventional medical doctor can look informed, modern, thoughtful and supportive to the patient who asks for natural medicine. Many medical doctors fear that practicing alternative medicine will lead to censure from their licensing body. But if they practice the complementary medicine contained herein they will be able to help their patients more effectively with no fear that they will hurt anyone. They are still the primary doctor, they can still make a diagnosis and prescribe drugs. Using these remedies they will find that the patient gets well faster with fewer side-effects.

Take this book when you go to see your doctor. After the doctor makes the diagnosis, look up the natural treatment herein. You might ask, "Would it be all right if I tried this along with what you are prescribing?" If the doctor gets angry and throws you out of the office, you can blame me. Sorry.

The remedies in this book can be used along with prescription drugs. In these situations, the amount of drug necessary to relieve symptoms will be small enough that side-effects will be minimal. All prescription drugs are toxic as they are foreign to the body and must be metabolized and eliminated. Conversely, the remedies in this book are safe and effective.

Dr. Stengler has condensed his years of medical study and treating patients into a clear and concise self-help book. Give it a try. You'll like it. Take charge of your body. "Whose body is it, after all?"

—Lendon H. Smith, MD
Author of *Feed Your Body Right* and *How To Raise A Healthy Child*

Preface

The first step in achieving and maintaining health is taking personal responsibility. Choosing a healthy lifestyle and choosing safer alternatives whenever possible and appropriate are a matter of education, choice and discipline. All of us who have found our path to a healthier way of life come by it differently. I've seen students and patients have significant life events where all of a sudden a spark was lit and there was no turning back after that. For most of us though, we need to be taught the basic steps, make slower changes, experiment, succeed and fail in our declarations and disciplines. Over time the momentum of the change in vitality in our bodies, minds and our emotions has a convincing effect. After that, we have a confidence in the effectiveness of our efforts and of natural methods of healing. This book offers you a resource to begin making changes towards a healthier lifestyle and safer, natural methods of health management.

With the help of this book, you can educate yourself, make changes, experiment and have successes with the benefits of natural healing methods. You just need to supply the discipline.

Be aware that naturopathic medicine and natural remedies are not appropriate for all people in all situations. Some women may, in fact, need hormone replacement therapy. There are appropriate times for surgeries. Judicious use of conventional medications are at times necessary and life saving. Educate yourself through resources not only supplied in this book, but by seeking out qualified, well-trained alternative practitioners. At times, it is also appropriate to seek out the expertise of a medical doctor who is also willing to respect your choices while at the same time offering you their best advice.

Ultimately, we are each responsible for our own health. Collectively, as we choose healthier habits, we will have healthier minds and bodies, healthier relationships with family members and friends, and a healthier planet on which to live.

—*Tori Hudson,* ND
Professor, National College of Naturopathic Medicine

Introduction

Natural medicine is quickly becoming an important component of the mainstream medical model. This growth in status has not come about as part of a fad—but of necessity! It is not surprising that a large percentage of the population seeks complementary forms of health care as our knowledge of these treatments expand. Society has learned that becoming proactive in one's health care can mean the difference between health and disease. Many of the so-called "wonder drugs" science has been proclaiming or searching for do not exist. In case after case I have seen health and vitality restored through natural treatments. The human body has a remarkable ability to heal. Often, all one needs is to maximize these amazing regenerative qualities. Better yet, following a preventative approach to health through diet, lifestyle and non-toxic therapies promotes health and reduces our susceptibility to illness.

Conventional medicine is excellent for life threatening situations such as broken bones or heart attacks. However, it does not serve to treat the underlying cause of most chronic illnesses. The beauty of natural medicine is that when properly applied it can prove useful in acute and chronic illnesses. Even when conventional medicine is being used for an acute or chronic illness, natural medicine can be used as an adjunct to accentuate healing.

This book has been written as a family guide to a natural and preventative approach to health. Many of the remedies in this book have been passed down through generations of physicians and natural healers. I have emphasized the therapies which I have found to be extremely effective with patients. The overwhelming majority of these strategies have the backing of extensive scientific research. There are different levels of prescribing and treating with natural medicine. At the most superficial level is the researcher who bases treatment plans on theory only. At the deepest level is the physician trained in natural medicine who uses both clinical experience and scientific research in tailoring treatment plans specifically to the individual. This guide provides a level of knowledge that could only be provided by a doctor that has actually used natural medicine to treat disease. To those searching for information on natural health care this is my gift to you.

Readers of this book are strongly encouraged to invest in preventative health care. Developing a relationship with a physician who has a strong foundation in natural medicine can be truly rewarding.

The Naturopathic Physician

Naturopathic physicians (NDs) are general practitioners trained as specialists in natural medicine. They are educated in the conventional medical sciences, but they are not orthodox medical doctors (MDs). Naturopathic physicians treat disease and restore health using therapies from the sciences of clinical nutrition, herbal medicine, homeopathy, physical medicine, exercise therapy, counseling, acupuncture, natural childbirth and hydrotherapy. They tailor these approaches to the needs of the individual patient. Naturopathic medicine is effective in treating most health problems, whether acute or chronic. Naturopathic physicians cooperate with all other branches of medical science, referring patients to other practitioners for diagnosis or treatment when appropriate.

In practice, naturopathic physicians perform physical examinations, laboratory testing, gynecological exams, nutritional and dietary assessments, metabolic analyses, allergy testing, X-ray examinations and other diagnostic tests. Treatments are tailored to the needs of the individual based on a cogent philosophy that acknowledges the patient as a participant.

The naturopathic physician has a Doctor of Naturopathic Medicine (ND) degree from a four-year, graduate-level naturopathic medical college. In states where they are regulated, naturopathic physicians must pass either a national or a state level board examination, and their actions are subject to review by a State (or Provincial) Board of Examiners.

Naturopathic physicians are the only primary-care physicians clinically trained in a wide variety of medical systems. Some of the natural therapies practiced by naturopathic physicians are:

Clinical Nutrition:
Nutrition and therapeutic use of foods have always been a cornerstone of naturopathic medicine. A growing body of scientific knowledge in this area is reflected in numerous professional journals of nutrition and dietary sciences, validating

the naturopathic approach to diet and nutrition. Many medical conditions can be treated as effectively with foods and nutritional supplements as they can by any other means, but with fewer complications and side-effects. Naturopathic physicians receive more than 140 classroom hours in clinical nutrition.

Homeopathic Medicine:
This powerful system of medicine is more than 200 years old, and is widely accepted in other countries (the Royal Family of England uses a homeopathic physician). Homeopathic medicines act to strengthen the body's innate immune response; they seldom have side-effects. Some conditions that conventional medicine has no effective treatment for respond well to homeopathy.

Botanical Medicine:
Many plant substances are powerful medicines. They are effective and safe when used properly, in the right dose and in the proper combinations with other herbs or treatments. A resurgence of scientific research in Europe and Asia is demonstrating that some plant substances are superior to synthetic drugs in clinical situations. Naturopathic doctors are trained in both the art and science of botanical medicine.

Physical Medicine:
In the last 100 years, various methods of applying treatments through the manipulation of the muscles, bones and spine have been developed. Naturopathic medicine has its own techniques, collectively known as naturopathic manipulative therapy. Physical medicine also includes but is not limited to physiotherapy using heat and cold, gentle electrical pulses, ultrasound, diathermy, hydrotherapy and exercise therapy.

Natural Childbirth:
Naturopathic physicians provide natural childbirth care in and out of hospital settings. They offer prenatal and postnatal care using the most modern diagnostic techniques. When natural childbirth is not medically indicated, because of high risk, patients are referred for appropriate care.

Oriental Medicine:
Naturopathic physicians are trained in the fundamentals of Oriental medicine and diagnosis, and many use acupuncture, acupressure and Oriental botanical medicine in their practices.

Counseling and Stress Management:
Mental attitudes and emotional states can be important elements in healing and disease. Naturopathic physicians are trained in various psychological techniques, including counseling, nutritional balancing, stress management, hypnotherapy, biofeedback and other methods.

Minor Surgery:
This includes repair of superficial wounds, removal of foreign bodies, cysts and other superficial masses, with local anesthesia as needed.

Principles of Naturopathic Medicine

The Healing Power of Nature:
Nature acts powerfully through the healing mechanisms in the body and mind to maintain and restore health. Naturopathic physicians work to rejuvenate and support these inherent healing systems when they have broken down by using methods, medicines and techniques that are in harmony with natural processes.

First Do No Harm:
Naturopathic physicians prefer non-invasive treatments which minimize the risks of harmful side-effects. They are trained to know which patients they can treat safely, and which ones they need to refer to other health care practitioners.

Find the Cause:
Every illness has an underlying cause, often in aspects of the lifestyle, diet or habits of the individual. A naturopathic physician is trained to find and remove the underlying cause of a disease.

Treat the Whole Person:
Health or disease come from a complex interaction of physical, emotional, dietary, genetic, environmental, lifestyle and other factors. Naturopathic physicians treat the whole person, taking all these factors into account.

Preventative Medicine:
The naturopathic approach to health care can prevent minor illnesses from developing into more serious or chronic degenerative diseases. Patients are taught principles for living a healthy life; by following these they can prevent major illnesses.

Doctor as Teacher:
The original Latin term for doctor was *docere* which means to teach. Educating patients how to become responsible for their own health is a fundamental goal of a naturopathic physician.

(*American Association of Naturopathic Physicians Brochure*)

Using This Guide

Each condition has a number of treatment options for you to choose from. Select one or a few that you can comfortably incorporate into your lifestyle.

● represents the primary and most effective choice
○ represents other helpful options

The easiest way to include several vitamin and mineral, or herbal remedies is to use a combination formula. The formula should include primary treatments (marked with ●) along with any number of the secondary treatments (marked with ○).

Note: Some products are only available in the U.S. and not in Canada. If you live in Canada and are unable to obtain these items, consider using a mail order company or shopping in the U.S.

Refer to the appendices at the back of the book for more detailed information on hydrotherapy, homeopathy, herbs, healthy diet, food allergies and sensitivities, and vitamins and minerals.

Acne

This condition is caused by overactive oil glands. Pores become blocked with accumulated bacteria and metabolic toxins and result in whiteheads, blackheads and inflamed pustules. Oil glands hypersecrete due to one or more of the following causes: improper diet, inefficient digestion, hormonal imbalance, nutritional deficiencies and genetics. It generally takes four to eight weeks of natural treatment to achieve improvement.

Nutrition

● Identify and eliminate **food allergies** and **sensitivities** (see *Appendix E*).
● **Reduce** sugar, fat, soda pop, alcohol and caffeine intake.

● **Increase water intake**—drink at least six to eight glasses of purified water daily.

○ Use **dairy alternatives** such as soy cheese, almond cheese, rice milk and soy milk.

○ Add **high fiber foods** to the diet such as apples, oat bran, broccoli, Brussels sprouts, cabbage, carrots, wholegrain flour and green leafy vegetables.

○ Take a **fiber supplement** that has psyllium seed husks as the base of the formula. Take as directed on bottle. Drink at least eight ounces of water with each dose.

○ **Avoid foods containing iodine** such as table salt because iodine can worsen acne formation.

Herbal

● **Flaxseed oil**—provides essential fatty acids for healthy skin. Take 2 capsules three times daily or 2 tablespoons daily.

● **Burdock root**—promotes detoxification. Take 1 capsule or 30 drops three times daily.

○ **Gentian root**—improves digestion. Take 1 capsule or 30 drops with meals.

○ **Berberis**—inhibits bacterial growth on skin and cleanses the blood. Take 1 capsule or 30 drops with meals.

○ **Milk thistle** (80% silymarin)—excellent for detoxification of the liver and skin. Take 250 mg daily or 30 drops with each meal.

○ **Angelica/Dong quai** (4:1 herb extract)—for hormone balancing, if needed. Take 1 capsule (125 mg) or 30 drops three times daily.

Vitamins and Minerals

● **Zinc**—promotes healthy skin regeneration. Take 50 mg daily (*if over age of fourteen*) with meals.

● **Copper**—a balancer for **zinc**. Take 3 mg daily with meals.

○ **Vitamin A**—specific for skin health. Take 25,000 IU daily with meals. (Consult with a physician when using high doses of Vitamin A.)

○ **Vitamin E**—for skin health. Take 800 IU daily with meals.

○ **Chromium**—imbalanced blood sugar levels may contribute to acne formation. Chromium acts to stabilize blood sugar levels. Take 400 mcg daily.

○ **Selenium**—specific for skin repair. Take daily total of 200 mcg.

Other

○ Wash with **unscented herbal soap** such as calendula or oatmeal. They are nonirritating and soothing to the skin.

○ Regular **exercise**—helps eliminate toxins from the body.

Alzheimer's

Symptoms of this condition include memory loss and deteri oration of thought processes, and can progress to the point of inability to complete daily activities. The naturopathic approach tries to prevent Alzheimer's from occurring if a family history is present. For individuals who already have this disease natural medicine can be used in an attempt to halt or slow its progression.

Nutrition

● It is advisable to follow a **plant-based diet** since red meat contains harmful saturated fat.

○ **Increase water intake**—drink at least six to eight glasses of purified water daily.

○ **Increase fiber**—add high fiber foods to the diet such as apples, oat bran, broccoli, Brussels sprouts, cabbage, carrots, wholegrain flour and green leafy vegetables.

○ **Avoid** refined sugar products, fatty foods, fried foods, margarine and dairy products.

○ Use **cold-pressed oils** such as extra-virgin olive oil or flaxseed oil. If you must fry, *never allow the oil to smoke*—use a medium heat and use extra-virgin olive oil or a heat resistant oil such as cold-pressed peanut or sesame oil. For baking at temperatures above 350°F use butter.

○ Eat **cold water fish** such as mackerel, herring and salmon because they contain essential fatty acids for artery health.

○ Eat **garlic, onions** and **legumes** liberally because they help detoxify the arteries.

○ **Avoid** caffeine, alcohol and tobacco products because they produce toxins.

Herbal

● **Ginkgo** (24% standardized extract)—increases circulation to the brain and improves neurotransmitter function. Take 1 capsule (80 mg) or 30 drops three times daily.

○ **Siberian ginseng** (0.4% eleutherosides)—helps stress adaption and improves mental alertness. Take 1 capsule (250 mg) or 30 drops three times daily.

Vitamins and Minerals

● **B complex**—take a 100 mg complex daily for nervous system health.

● **Vitamin B12**—involved with proper function of the nervous system. Talk to your physician about injections of this vitamin.

○ **Coenzyme Q10**—a potent antioxidant that improves oxygenation in the cells. Take 200 mg daily.

○ **Zinc**—helps prevent degeneration of the nervous system. Take 50 mg daily with 3 mg of **copper**.

○ **High potency multi-vitamin without iron**—take one daily with a meal.

○ **Folic acid**—involved with proper function of the nervous system. Talk to your physician about injections of this vitamin.

○ **Acetyl-l-carnitine**—believed to enhance brain metabolism. Take 500 mg twice daily.

Other

● Consider **homeopathy** from a qualified practitioner.

○ **Lecithin**—used by the brain to make the neurotransmitter acetylcholine. Take 5 g three times daily.

○ **Avoid aluminum** and **silicon** which may play a role in causing this illness. These substances are commonly found in antacids, antiperspirants, cooking pots and water supplies.

○ Consider **chelation therapy** if there is a history of heavy metal exposure.

○ **DHEA**—may have a protective effect on brain cells. Dosage can range from 25 to 300 mg (talk to your physician about its use).

○ Consider **acupuncture** from a qualified practitioner.

○ **Salmon oil**—supplies omega-3 fatty acids for nerve and artery health. Take 2 capsules (1,000 mg each) twice daily.

Anemia

This condition refers to a deficiency of red blood cells or hemoglobin (the component of red blood cells that contains iron). Since these cells carry oxygen throughout the body a deficiency can result in fatigue, pallor and weakness. There are different types and causes of anemia. The main types are iron, B12 and folic acid deficiency anemias which are determined by a blood test. Other clinical evaluation may be necessary to determine the cause of the anemia.

Nutrition

○ **Avoid coffee** and **tea** which can interfere with iron absorption and deplete the body of B vitamins.

○ **Blackstrap molasses**—contains iron and B vitamins. Adults should take 1 tablespoon twice daily and children should take 1 teaspoon twice daily.

○ **Brewer's yeast**—supplies many minerals, especially B vitamins. Take 1 teaspoon twice daily.

○ **Organic calf liver**—contains iron as well as B vitamins. The recommended portion is four ounces three times weekly.

○ **Green leafy vegetables**—consume daily for mineral content.

Herbal

● **Rumex**—helps with iron absorption. Take 1 capsule or 30 drops three times daily for at least one month.

● **Chlorophyll**—contains the precursors necessary for blood production. Take 1 tablespoon, 3 capsules or 3 tablets daily.

○ **Gentian root**—improves stomach function so that the nutrients are better absorbed. Take 1 to 2 capsules or 20 to 30 drops tincture at the beginning of each meal.

○ **Stinging nettle**—high in mineral content. Take 1 capsule or 30 drops three times daily for at least one month.

Vitamins and Minerals

Supplementation depends on the type of anemia:

○ **Iron deficiency**—for mild anemia I do not find iron supplementation necessary. The other mentioned treatments are usually sufficient. For moderate to severe iron deficiency I recommend 30 to 50 mg daily of **iron**. **Vitamin C with bioflavonoids** helps with iron absorption. Take 1,000 mg with each dose of iron supplementation with meals.

○ **Folic acid deficiency**—take 800 mcg daily.

○ **B12 deficiency**—take 1 mg daily.

Note: Folic acid and B12 are utilized more efficiently when given by injection. Talk to a physician about this technique.

○ **High potency multi-vitamin**—take daily.

Other

● **Homeopathic *Ferrum phos* 6x** and ***Calc phos* 6x**—helps to build up the red blood cells. Take a dose of each three times daily away from food or drink for at least two months.

○ **Liver glandular extract**—builds up the red blood cells.

○ **Chinese herbal medicine** can be very effective in resolving different types of anemia. See a qualified practitioner.

Angina

This condition refers to chest pain that results from an inadequate supply of blood to the heart. A sharp or squeezing pain is often felt after physical exertion. Contributing factors include atherosclerosis, high blood pressure and stress. It is these factors that need to be addressed in order to treat the cause of this serious condition.

Nutrition

- It is advisable to follow a **plant-based diet** since red meat contains harmful saturated fat.
- ○ **Increase fiber**—add high fiber foods to the diet such as apples, oat bran, broccoli, Brussels sprouts, cabbage, carrots, wholegrain flour and green leafy vegetables.
- ○ **Increase water intake**—drink at least six to eight glasses of purified water daily.
- ○ Use **cold-pressed oils** such as extra-virgin olive oil or flaxseed oil. If you must fry, *never allow the oil to smoke*— use a medium heat and use extra-virgin olive oil or a heat resistant oil such as cold-pressed peanut or sesame oil. For baking at temperatures above 350°F use butter.
- ○ Eat **cold water fish** such as mackerel, herring and salmon because they contain essential fatty acids for artery health.
- ○ Eat **garlic, onions** and **legumes** liberally because they help detoxify the arteries.
- ○ **Avoid** caffeine, alcohol and tobacco products.
- ○ **Limit sodium** intake.
- ○ **Avoid** artificial sweeteners and food preservatives as much as possible—consume fresh foods.

Herbal

- **Hawthorn** (1.8% vitexin-4'rhamnoside)—increases blood flow to the heart and reduces blood pressure. Take 250 mg three times daily.
- **Cactus**—improves the contractive ability of the heart. Take 10 drops of extract twice daily.
- ○ **Ginkgo** (24% standardized extract)—improves circulation through the cardiovascular system. Take 1 capsule (40 mg) or 30 drops three times daily.

○ **Flaxseed oil**—supplies essential fatty acids for artery health. Take 1 to 2 tablespoons daily.

○ **Garlic**—improves circulation as well as reducing cholesterol and fats in the blood. Take 2 capsules daily or a daily total of standardized allicin content of 5,000 mcg.

○ **Bromelain**—breaks down plaques in the blood vessels. Take 500 mg three times daily between meals.

Vitamins and Minerals

● **Coenzyme Q10**—a nutrient for efficient heart contraction and oxygenation of heart tissue. Take 100 mg twice daily.

○ **Magnesium**—used by the heart for muscle contraction. Take 250 mg twice daily.

○ **Vitamin E**—potent antioxidant for the heart. Take 400 IU twice daily.

○ **L-Carnitine**—used by the heart muscle to efficiently convert fatty acids to energy. Take 500 mg three times daily.

○ **B complex**—supplies complex of vitamins for energy and stress. Take a 50 mg complex once daily.

Other

○ **Stress relaxation** techniques—exercise and mental imagery.

○ Consider **chelation therapy** from a qualified practitioner.

○ **Homeopathic *Cactus* 30C**—take a dose as needed for squeezing pains in the chest (do not replace the use of pharmaceutical medication, but use in combination with— discuss with your physician).

○ Consider **acupuncture** from a qualified practitioner.

○ **Salmon oil**—supplies omega-3 fatty acids for nerve and artery health. Take 2 capsules (1,000 mg each) two to three times daily.

Anxiety

This condition refers to an uneasiness of the mind that may be accompanied by physical symptoms such as sweating and increased pulse rate. Acute attacks, also known as "panic attacks," can occur at any time and produce tremendous feelings of anxiety and fear. Biochemical imbalances such as hypoglycemia can be responsible for anxiety. As well, mental and emotional factors need to be explored and treated for long-term improvement.

Nutrition

○ **Avoid** stimulants that contain **caffeine**—coffee, black tea, soda pop and chocolate.
○ **Limit refined sugar** intake and use honey as a sweetener.
○ Eat **smaller meals more frequently** throughout the day. This helps balance blood sugar and decreases anxiety symptoms.
○ Identify and eliminate **food sensitivities** (see *Appendix E*).

Herbal

The following herbs act to calm and nourish the nervous system:

● **Valerian**—take 1 to 2 capsules (100 to 300 mg each) or 30 to 60 drops three times daily.
● **Passion flower**—take 1 capsule (100 mg) or 30 drops three times daily.
● **St. John's wort** (0.3% hypercin)—take 1 capsule or 30 drops three times daily.
○ **Avena sativa**—take 1 to 2 capsules or 30 to 60 drops three times daily.
○ **Chamomile**—drink 1 cup of tea three times daily.
○ **Kava kava**—take 1 capsule (100 mg) or 30 drops three times daily.

Vitamins and Minerals

○ **B complex**—these vitamins are used in the energy pathways and become depleted with stress. Take a 50 mg complex daily.
○ **Calcium** and **magnesium**—these nutrients are necessary for relaxation of the nervous system. Take 500 to 1,000 mg of each daily with meals.

○ **Chromium**—balances blood sugar levels. Take 200 mcg twice daily.

Other

● **Stress reduction** techniques—exercise, yoga, t'ai chi and mental imagery.

● **Homeopathic Rescue Remedy**—take 5 drops three times daily or immediately when anxiety symptoms begin.

○ **Homeopathic *Kali phos* 6x**—works to calm and tonify the nervous system. Take a dose three times daily.

Arthritis (Osteoarthritis)

This is the most common form of arthritis where degenerative changes take place in the joint tissue. Over a period of time the joints become stiff and painful and loss of mobility may occur. Natural therapies can be effective in reversing this degenerative process.

Nutrition

The following foods can increase inflammation:
○ **Avoid caffeine**—coffee, tea, chocolate and soda pop.
○ **Avoid** alcohol, tobacco and sugar products.
○ **Avoid** tomatoes, eggplant, peppers (not black pepper) and potatoes.

● Identify and eliminate **food sensitivities** (see *Appendix E*).
○ Eat plenty of fruit—specifically **cherries**.
○ Eat **dairy alternatives** such as soy cheese, almond cheese, rice milk or soy milk.
○ **Fresh fruit** and **vegetable juices** are excellent.

Herbal

● **Licorice root** (12% glycyrrhizin)—has potent anti-inflammatory effects. Take 100 mg three times daily.

- **Black cohosh** (4:1 extract)—relieves muscle and joint pain. Take 25 mg three times daily.
- ○ **Flaxseed oil**—contains essential fatty acids that help reduce inflammation. Take 1 to 2 tablespoons daily.
- ○ **Bromelain**—useful for acute flare-ups of arthritic pain. Take 500 mg three times daily on an empty stomach.
- ○ **Cat's claw** (3% alkaloids)—is a potent anti-inflammatory. Take 200 mg three times daily.
- ○ **Ginger root**—increases circulation, decreases inflammation and helps in proper absorption of nutrients. Take 1 to 2 capsules or 30 to 60 drops three times daily.
- ○ **Yucca extract** (40% saponins)—known for its natural anti-inflammatory effects. Take 1 capsule (1 g) or 30 drops three times daily.

Vitamins and Minerals

- **Glucosamine sulfate**—regenerates joint tissues. Take 500 mg three times daily for a minimum of two months.
- **Chondroitin sulfate**—has a regenerating effect on joint tissues. Take 500 mg three times daily for a minimum of two months.
- ○ **Multi-vitamin without iron**—for general health enhancement. Take one daily.
- ○ **Vitamin C with bioflavonoids**—builds up connective tissues in body and protects against tissue damage. Take 1,000 mg three times daily.
- ○ **Vitamin E**—protects against joint damage. Take a total of 400 to 800 IU daily.
- ○ **Grape seed extract (PCO)** (95% leucoanthocyanins)—is a powerful natural anti-inflammatory. Take 50 mg three times daily.

Other

- **Constitutional hydrotherapy**—see *Appendix A*.
- Consider **acupuncture** and **Chinese herbal medicine**.
- Consider **homeopathy** from a qualified practitioner.

○ **Betaine HCl**—improves stomach digestion and absorption of minerals. Take 1 to 2 tablets with meals.

○ **DHEA**—may help to slow down or reverse tissue degradation. Take 25 to 100 mg daily (talk to your physician about its use).

○ **Exercise**—promotes circulation and decreases inflammation. Aerobic exercise such as swimming and walking are excellent. Exercise for half an hour four to six times weekly.

○ **Glandular extracts** of connective tissue—used to build up joint tissues. Take 1 capsule three times daily.

○ **Homeopathic** *Calc fluor* **6x**—specific for connective tissue health. One dose three times daily.

○ **Homeopathic** *Calc phos* **6x**—specific for bone health. Take one dose three times daily.

Asthma

Asthma is an allergic condition that results in episodes of wheezing, coughing and shortness of breath. Severe attacks can be life threatening and require emergency medical attention. Overall health must be enhanced so that the respiratory system is not so hypersensitive.

Nutrition

Many studies have shown that elimination of **food allergies** and **sensitivities** can greatly improve this condition. My clinical experience has shown this to be true. See *Appendix E*.

● Avoid dairy products, eggs, citrus fruit, nuts, salt, large amounts of red meat and wheat products.

● Avoid foods or products that contain artificial preservatives.

○ Eat **large amounts** of vegetables, rice, non-citrus fruit, fish, chicken and small amounts of red meat.

○ Eat **cold water fish** such as mackerel, herring and salmon. They contain essential fatty acids which may reduce bronchial inflammation.

○ Fresh juicing can be extremely valuable. Drink **fresh, organic juices** daily.

○ Consider a three day **juice fast** to detoxify the body.

Herbal

- **Licorice root** (12% glycyrrhizin)—is a natural anti-inflammatory. Take 2 capsules or 60 drops three times daily.
- ○ **Mullein**—soothes the respiratory tract. Take 2 capsules or 60 drops four times daily.
- ○ **Gentian root**—stimulates stomach function to help absorb nutrients more efficiently and reduces reactions to foods that may trigger attacks. Take 2 capsules or 60 drops with meals.
- ○ **Ephedra**—formulas containing ephedra are useful on a short-term basis to help reduce asthma symptoms.

Vitamins and Minerals

The following vitamins are useful in preventing asthma reactions:
- **Quercitin**—take 500 mg three times daily.
- **Magnesium** and **calcium**—take 500 mg of each daily.
- **Vitamin B12**—take 1 mg daily. It is useful to have B12 injected by your physician.
- ○ **B complex**—take a 50 mg complex twice daily. It is useful to have B vitamins injected by your physician.
- ○ **Vitamin C with bioflavonoids**—take 1,000 mg three times daily in divided doses.
- ○ **High potency multi-vitamin**—take once daily with meals.

Other

- **Homeopathy** from a qualified practitioner is very effective.
- **Acupuncture** from a qualified practitioner is very effective.
- ○ **Betaine HCl**—taken with meals helps to ensure proper digestion of food. Many asthmatics have been shown to be deficient in hydrochloric acid which in turn leads to food reactions and vitamin deficiencies such as B12.
- ○ **DHEA**—supports the body's anti-inflammatory hormones. Talk to your physician about its use.
- ○ **Pregnenolone**—supports the body's anti-inflammatory hormones. Talk to your physician about its use.

○ **Stress reduction** techniques such as mental imagery, hypnosis and counseling are helpful.

○ **Avoid** known environmental pollutants (especially smoke) and allergens. Install air filter (HEPA) in home.

Atherosclerosis

Refers to the plaque build-up of fat, cholesterol and calcium inside the artery walls. This impedes blood flow throughout the heart and other areas of the body. As this plaque build-up advances, one becomes susceptible to serious medical conditions such as stroke and heart attack. Atherosclerosis can be caused by, or may lead to, high blood pressure. Diet and lifestyle changes have been shown to reverse this degenerative condition.

Nutrition

● **Increase fiber**—add high fiber foods to the diet such as apples, oat bran, broccoli, Brussels sprouts, cabbage, carrots, wholegrain flour and green leafy vegetables.

○ It is advisable to follow a **plant-based diet** since red meat contains harmful saturated fat.

○ **Increase water intake**—drink at least six to eight glasses of purified water daily.

○ Take a **fiber supplement** that has psyllium seed husks as the base of the formula. Take as directed on bottle. Drink at least eight ounces of water with each dose.

○ **Avoid** refined sugar products, fatty foods, margarine, alcohol, caffeine and dairy products.

○ Use **cold-pressed oils** such as extra-virgin olive oil or flaxseed oil. If you must fry, *never allow the oil to smoke*— use a medium heat and use extra-virgin olive oil or a heat resistant oil such as cold-pressed peanut or sesame oil. For baking at temperatures above 350°F use butter.

○ Eat **cold water fish** such as mackerel, herring and salmon because they contain essential fatty acids for artery health.

○ Eat **garlic, onions** and **legumes** liberally.

Herbal

- **Gugulipid**—decreases high cholesterol and triglyceride levels. Take 500 mg of gugulipid (with a guggulsterone content of 25 mg) three times daily.
- **Ginkgo** (24% standardized extract)—improves circulation. Take 1 capsule (60 mg) or 30 drops three times daily.
- **Garlic**—reduces cholesterol and detoxifies the arteries. Take 2 capsules or 30 drops three times daily or a daily total of standardized allicin content of 5,000 mcg.
- ○ **Cayenne**—improves circulation in the arteries and reduces cholesterol. Take as directed on container.
- ○ **Ginger**—improves circulation and reduces fats and cholesterol. Take 1 capsule or 30 drops three times daily.
- ○ **Bromelain**—breaks down plaques in the blood vessels. Take 500 mg three times daily between meals.
- ○ **Flaxseed oil**—take 1 tablespoon daily for essential fatty acids.

Vitamins and Minerals

The following vitamins protect against artery damage:

- **Coenzyme Q10**—protective effect on the cardiovascular system. Take 60 mg three times daily.
- **High potency multi-vitamin without iron**—take on a daily basis with a meal.
- **Niacin** (inositol hexaniacinate form)—decreases cholesterol and improves circulation. Take 500 mg three times daily.
- ○ **B complex**—take a 50 mg complex daily.
- ○ **Vitamin E**—take a total of 800 IU daily.
- ○ **Chromium**—take 400 mcg daily.
- ○ **Vitamin C with bioflavonoids**—take 3,000 to 5,000 mg daily in divided doses.
- ○ **Lecithin**—take 5 to 10 mg daily.

Other

- Consider **chelation therapy** from a qualified practitioner.
- ○ **Avoid smoking**.

○ **Exercise** on a regular basis.
○ **High blood pressure** needs to be addressed to prevent further plaque formation (see *High Blood Pressure* section).
○ **Salmon oil**—supplies omega-3 fatty acids for artery health. Take 2 capsules (1,000 mg each) two to three times daily.
○ **Chinese herbal medicine** from a qualified practitioner.

Athlete's Foot

This is an opportunistic fungal infection that grows on the skin of the foot and sometimes the toenails. Symptoms can in-clude itching, burning, and scaling or cracking of the skin. It is important to detoxify the body from the inside out so that the skin is less susceptible to fungal infection.

Nutrition

● **Avoid refined sugars**. Use honey as a sweetener.
○ **Avoid caffeine**—coffee, tea, chocolate and soda pop.
○ **Avoid** alcohol and tobacco products.
○ Eat **dairy alternatives** such as soy cheese, almond cheese, rice milk or soy milk.
○ **Fresh fruit** and **vegetable juices**—make your own daily.

Herbal

● **Tea tree oil**—apply with a Q-tip to the infected area twice daily for a minimum of six weeks.
○ **Garlic**—has antifungal properties. Take 5,000 mcg of standardized allicin content daily.
○ **Cat's claw** (3% alkaloids)—immune stimulant. Take 200 mg three times daily.
○ **Calendula tincture**—apply topically every day to cracks in skin for rapid healing.
○ **Burdock root**—acts as a detoxifier. Take 1 to 2 capsules or 30 to 60 drops three times daily.

Vitamins and Minerals

○ **Vitamin C with bioflavonoids**—enhances immune system function. Take 3,000 mg daily in divided doses.

○ **Zinc**—essential for wound and skin healing. Take 30 mg daily **with** 3 mg of **copper.**

○ **Chromium**—balances blood sugar which is often a problem in this condition. Take 200 mcg daily.

○ **High potency multi-vitamin without iron**—take daily to correct nutritional deficiencies.

Other

○ Consider a three to five day **juice fast.**

○ **Keep infected area dry.** Change socks often.

Athletic Performance Enhancement

Athletes involved in high intensity training require a comprehensive natural support program. Athletes have a greater demand for supplementation to aid recovery from training. The following Natural Physician Performance Enhancement Program is a guideline for athletes or those in training. It has three main objectives:

• improve athletic performance
• reduce the amount of time needed to recover from training
• prevent mental and physical burn-out from long-term training

Nutrition

● It is important to **replace electrolytes, protein** and **carbohydrates** within half an hour after a training session. Recovery drinks can be useful.

○ **Eat three to five meals daily. High quality protein** is important for muscle and tissue repair. Quality sources of protein include fish, turkey breast, chicken breast, eggs, beans and soy products. **Complex carbohydrates** should be eaten as a main energy source.

○ **Increase fiber**—add high fiber foods to the diet such as apples, oat bran, broccoli, Brussels sprouts, cabbage, carrots, wholegrain flour and green leafy vegetables.

○ **Increase water intake**—drink at least six to eight glasses of purified water daily. Avoid water containing chlorine.

○ **Avoid** refined sugar products, fatty foods, margarine, alcohol, caffeine and dairy products.

○ Use **cold-pressed oils** such as extra-virgin olive oil or flaxseed oil. If you must fry, *never allow the oil to smoke*—use a medium heat and use extra-virgin olive oil or a heat resistant oil such as cold-pressed peanut or sesame oil. For baking at temperatures above 350°F use butter.

○ Eat **cold water fish** such as mackerel, herring and salmon because they contain essential fatty acids for artery health.

○ Eat **garlic** and **onions** liberally as they help detoxify the arteries.

○ **Fresh fruit** and **vegetable juices** are excellent.

Herbal

● **Siberian ginseng** (0.4% eleutherosides)—an excellent herb to help the body recover from physical as well as mental stress. Take 250 mg or 30 drops two to three times daily.

○ **American ginseng** (panax ginseng)—helps the body deal with physical and mental stress. Also helps to stimulate energy levels. Take 1 to 2 capsules (100 mg each) or 30 to 60 drops three times daily for four weeks on then two weeks off. Repeat this cycle as needed.

○ **Ginkgo** (24% standardized extract)—increases circulation and improves mental concentration. Take 1 capsule (60 mg) or 30 drops three times daily.

○ **Licorice root** (12% glycyrrhizin)—is a natural anti-inflammatory and nourishes the adrenal (stress) glands. Take 1 capsule or 30 drops three times daily.

○ **Milk thistle** (80% silymarin)—assists liver in detoxification. Take 150 mg capsule or 30 to 45 drops three times daily.

○ **Blue-green algae**—supplies amino acids and trace minerals necessary for tissue repair. Take as directed on container.

Vitamins and Minerals

● **High potency multi-vitamin without iron**—to ensure a base level of necessary vitamins and minerals. Take one daily with a meal.

● **Coenzyme Q10**—important for cell oxygenation and energy production. Take 60 to 120 mg daily.

○ **Vitamin C with bioflavonoids**—supports the immune system, repairs connective tissue and supports the stress glands. Take 3,000 mg daily in divided doses.

○ **Grape seed extract (PCO)**—repairs connective tissue and increases the effectiveness of **vitamin C**. Take 50 to 100 mg daily.

○ **L-Carnitine**—aids body in efficiently utilizing fatty acids for energy. Take 500 mg daily with meals.

○ **Chromium**—regulates blood sugar and promotes lean muscle mass. Take 200 mcg daily.

○ **Calcium**—used for muscle and nerve function. Maintains bone development. Take 1,000 mg daily with a meal.

○ **Magnesium**—used for muscle and nerve function. Maintains bone development. Take 1,000 mg daily with a meal.

Other

● **Creatine**—research shows this supplement helps the muscles to store more energy and to maintain or increase lean muscle mass. An average dosage is 3 to 5 g an hour before and immediately after training (dosage varies depending on body weight and training intensity).

○ **Salmon oil**—supplies omega-3 fatty acids for cardiovascular health. Take 2 capsules (1,000 mg each) two to three times daily.

○ **Homeopathic *Arnica* 30C**—use for acute trauma from training. Take a dose twice daily until tissue soreness is gone.

○ **Homeopathic *Rhus tox* 30C**—to be used for tissue damage and stiffness due to overexertion. Take a dose twice daily until stiffness is gone.

○ Homeopathic *Lactic acid* **6x**—this remedy can be taken during training to help eliminate waste products and decrease recovery time. Take a dose twice daily while you are training.

○ Homeopathic *Nat phos* **6x**—another remedy that can be taken during training to help eliminate waste products and decrease recovery time. Take a dose twice daily while you are training.

The following therapies help to promote recuperation from training:

● **Massage** from a qualified practitioner.
● **Acupuncture** from a qualified practitioner.
○ **Constitutional hydrotherapy**—see *Appendix A*.
○ **Spinal manipulation** or **chiropractic** from a qualified practitioner.
○ **Mental imagery** to relax and envision training and competing successfully.

Bites and Stings

Minor insect bites and bee stings can be relieved with natural therapies. Any animal bites and signs of infection or shock (weakness, dizziness, difficulty breathing, severe swelling or nausea) should receive immediate medical attention.

Herbal

● **Calendula**—promotes healing of tissue and is a natural antiseptic. Apply with a cotton ball to affected area four to five times daily.

Vitamins and Minerals

○ **Vitamin C with bioflavonoids**—a natural anti-inflammatory that reduces swelling and pain. Take 1,000 mg daily in three divided doses.

Other

- **Charcoal poultice**—used to adsorb toxins that are left by a sting or bite. Dissolve 2 activated charcoal tablets in four ounces of water, then spread this charcoal paste over a paper towel until it is well moistened. Cover the affected skin with the paper towel then with a piece of plastic. Secure this poultice with a bandage.
- **Homeopathic *Apis* 30C**—relieves pain and swelling of bee stings. Take a dose every half-hour until symptoms subside.
- **Homeopathic *Ledum* 30C**—used to help relieve pain and swelling of mosquito bites. Take a dose every half-hour until symptoms subside.

Black Eye

Trauma to the tissue of the eye and surrounding area results in broken blood vessels and results in dark discoloration. Any internal eye damage should be under the care of a medical professional.

Nutrition

- **Eat plenty of fruit** to help supply bioflavonoids and other ingredients necessary for the healing of bruises.
- **Avoid** sugar products as they slow down the repair process.

Herbal

- **Bromelain**—heals damaged tissue. Take 500 mg three times daily between meals.
- **Arnica oil**—heals damaged tissue. Apply to bruised area. Be careful to avoid getting any oil into the eyes or on broken skin.

Vitamins and Minerals

- **Vitamin C with bioflavonoids**—take 1,000 mg three times daily for blood vessel and tissue repair.

Other

- **Apply an ice pack** to the eye **immediately** after injury to reduce pain and swelling.
- After twenty-four hours, apply **alternating hot and cold compresses** to the eye.
- **Homeopathic *Arnica* 30C**—take a dose of the medicine every two hours for one day. This is an extremely effective treatment for healing traumatized tissue.

Boils

These skin lesions occur when the hair follicle becomes infected and pus forms. Boils are red and tender and may be accompanied by fever. Boils that occur in clusters are called a carbuncle. Generally pus builds up and comes to a head that opens up and drains. Severely infected boils require medical attention.

Nutrition

- **Avoid excessive amounts of sugar** as it can lower immune function and promote infection.
- Chronic boils may be related to **food allergies** and **sensitivities**. Offending foods should be identified and removed from the diet (see *Appendix E*).
- A three day **juice fast** may be helpful in detoxifying the skin and accelerating the healing of the boils.

Herbal

- **Goldenseal**—fights infections. Take 2 capsules or 60 drops four times daily. Also, apply goldenseal **topically**—make a poultice (mix 1 tablespoon of goldenseal powder with an egg white to form a paste) and apply it to the boil.
- **Echinacea** (4% echinacosides and 0.7% flavonoids)—fights infections and detoxifies the blood. Take 2 capsules (250 mg each) or 60 drops four times daily.

Vitamins and Minerals

The following vitamins stimulate the immune system and fight infections:

○ **Vitamin C with bioflavonoids**—1,000 mg three times daily.
○ **Beta-carotene**—take 100,000 IU daily.
○ **Zinc**—take 30 mg daily **with** 3 mg of **copper**.

Other

● Apply **hot wet cloths** to boil to bring it to a head and let the pus drain. Seek medical intervention if infection persists.
● **Homeopathic *Silicea* 6x and *Hepar sulph* 3x**—take a dose of each remedy three times daily until the boil resolves.

Bronchitis

Bronchitis is a viral respiratory tract infection that invades the bronchial tubes (breathing passageways). This irritation produces symptoms such as fever, coughing and chest pain. Prompt treatment can prevent pneumonia from developing.

Nutrition

○ **Avoid dairy products** because they are known to increase mucus formation in certain people. Use dairy alternatives such as soy cheese, almond cheese, rice milk or soy milk.
○ **Avoid sugar** because it can lower immune function.
○ Identify and eliminate **food sensitivities** if chronic bronchitis is a problem (see *Appendix E*).

Herbal

● **Goldenseal**—fights infections. Take 2 capsules or 60 drops every two hours for acute infections.
● **Cherry bark**—used for coughs and respiratory infections. Take 2 capsules or 60 drops every two hours for acute infections.

- **Echinacea** (4% echinacosides and 0.7% flavonoids)—fights infections. Take 2 capsules (250 mg each) or 60 drops every two hours for acute infections.
- ○ **Marshmallow root**—relieves pain of respiratory tract. Take 2 capsules or 60 drops every two hours for acute infections.
- ○ **Garlic capsules**—an immune stimulant. Take 2 capsules of 5,000 mcg standardized allicin content three times daily.
- ○ **Onion cough syrup**—boil five chopped onions with half a cup of honey, cook at low heat for two hours and strain. Drink warm, one cup every one to two hours.

Vitamins and Minerals

- **Vitamin C with bioflavonoids**—1,000 mg every three hours.
- ○ **Beta-carotene**—100,000 IU daily.
- ○ **Zinc**—50 mg daily.

Other

- **Constitutional hydrotherapy**—an excellent treatment to relieve congestion of the bronchial tubes. See *Appendix A*.
- ○ **Avoid smoke** and other **airborne pollutants** that irritate the respiratory passageway.
- ○ **Homeopathy** from a qualified practitioner.
- ○ **Chinese herbal medicine** from a qualified practitioner.

Bruises

Damage to the tissues results in broken blood vessels and pooling of blood. As a result pain, swelling and black-blue discoloration occur. Chronic tendency to bruising may be related to deficiencies such as iron or vitamin C. It may also be caused by underlying diseases and should be investigated by a medical professional.

Nutrition

- ○ Eat plenty of **fruit** to help supply bioflavonoids and other ingredients necessary for the healing of bruises.

Herbal

- **Bromelain**—an excellent herbal extract for the healing of bruises. Take 500 mg three times daily on an empty stomach.
- ○ **Arnica tincture**—heals damaged tissue. Apply to bruise topically. *Do not use if skin is broken.*

Vitamins and Minerals

- **Vitamin C with bioflavonoids**—1,000 mg three times daily.
- ○ **High potency multi-vitamin**—take daily with a meal to ensure against nutritional deficiencies.
- ○ **Vitamin E**—helps repair damaged tissue. Take 400 IU daily.

Other

- **Homeopathic *Arnica* 30C**—for acute bruises. An extremely effective treatment for this condition. Take a dose twice daily until bruising pain is gone.
- ○ **Homeopathic *Ferrum phos* 6x**—take a dose three times daily for chronic tendency to bruise.
- ○ **Apply an ice pack** to the bruised area **immediately** after injury to reduce pain and swelling.
- ○ After 24 hours, **apply alternating hot and cold compresses**.
- ○ Consider **Chinese herbal medicine** from a qualified practitioner.
- ○ **Anemia** may be the cause of chronic bruising (see *Anemia* section).

Burns

Minor burns may be treated effectively at home. Burns that become infected or occur in highly visible areas (face) should receive medical attention.

Nutrition

- ○ **Increase protein** in diet by including fish, meat or blue-green algae to promote tissue healing.

○ Drink large amounts of **purified water.**

Herbal

● **Aloe vera**—soothes skin. Apply to burn four to five times daily.
○ **Calendula**—heals skin. Apply tincture liberally to burn four to five times daily.

Vitamins and Minerals

● **Vitamin E gel**—apply gel to unbroken burned skin three times daily to promote healing and reduce scarring.
● **Zinc**—promotes regeneration of damaged tissue. Take 50 mg daily until burn is healed.
○ **Copper**—used in conjunction with **zinc**. Take 3 mg daily until burn is healed.
○ **Vitamin C with bioflavonoids**—heals tissue. Take 1,000 mg three times daily.
○ **High potency multi-vitamin without iron**—take daily to accelerate wound healing.
○ **Vitamin A**—heals skin. Take 25,000 IU daily until burn is healed.

Other

● **Homeopathic *Cantharis* 30C**—take a dose every half-hour until pain subsides.
○ **Homeopathic *Causticum* 30C**—useful for chemical burns. Take a dose every half-hour until pain subsides.

Bursitis

A condition where the bursa (thin sacs that secrete a fluid to lubricate joint tissue) become inflamed, causing severe pain during movement. This occurs from trauma and overuse of the joints. The shoulder joint is the most common site for bursitis.

Nutrition

Avoid the following foods which can increase inflammation:
○ **Avoid caffeine**—coffee, tea, chocolate and soda pop.
○ **Avoid** alcohol, tobacco and sugar products.
○ **Avoid** tomatoes, eggplant, peppers (not black pepper) and potatoes.

○ Eat plenty of **fruit**—specifically cherries.
○ Eat **dairy alternatives** such as soy cheese, almond cheese, rice milk or soy milk.
○ **Fresh fruit** and **vegetable juices** are excellent.
○ Identify and eliminate **food sensitivities** as they can aggravate this condition (see *Appendix E*).
○ Consider a three day **juice fast** to reduce toxicity and inflammation in the body and joints.

Herbal

● **Bromelain**—a natural anti-inflammatory. Take 500 mg three times daily between meals.
○ **Devil's claw**—also known for its anti-inflammatory effects. Take one capsule or 30 drops three times daily.
○ **Flaxseed oil**—essential fatty acids help reduce pain and inflammation. Take 1 to 2 tablespoons daily.

Vitamins and Minerals

○ **Vitamin B12**—have 1 mg injected intramuscularly by your physician every day for ten days. Then take as needed to keep the inflammation stabilized.
○ **Grape seed extract (PCO)**—promotes healing of joint and connective tissue. Take 100 mg daily.
○ **Vitamin E**—a natural anti-inflammatory. Take 800 IU daily.
○ **Calcium and magnesium**—take 1,000 mg of each daily for proper connective tissue repair.
○ **Vitamin C with bioflavonoids**—decreases inflammation and strengthens connective tissue. Take 1,000 mg four times daily.

Other

○ **Glucosamine sulfate**—an anti-inflammatory and used to build and repair joint tissue. Take 500 mg three times daily.

○ **Salmon oil**—supplies omega-3 fatty acids that reduce pain and inflammation. Take 2 capsules (1,000 mg each) twice daily.

○ **Homeopathic *Ferrum phos* 6x**—decreases inflammation. Take a dose three times daily.

○ Consider **spinal manipulation** or **chiropractic** by a qualified practitioner.

○ Consider **physiotherapy** from a qualified practitioner.

○ Consider **acupuncture** from a qualified practitioner.

Cancer

This term refers to the abnormal growth of cells. There are many known causes of cancer such as nutritional deficiencies, environmental pollution, stress and genetic abnormalities. Natural medicine should be an integral part of cancer treatment and is often used in combination with conventional therapies. It is important for the underlying cause to be addressed when creating a treatment program with your physician.

Nutrition

○ Follow a **plant-based diet** since red meat contains harmful saturated fat. Increase intake of fruit and vegetables.

○ **Increase fiber**—add high fiber foods to the diet such as apples, oat bran, broccoli, Brussels sprouts, cabbage, carrots, wholegrain flour and green leafy vegetables.

○ Take a **fiber supplement** that has psyllium seed husks as the base of the formula. Take as directed on container. Drink at least eight ounces of water with each dose.

○ **Increase water intake**—drink at least six to eight glasses of purified water daily.

○ **Strictly avoid** refined sugar products, fatty foods, fried foods, margarine, alcohol, caffeine and dairy products.

○ Use **cold-pressed oils** such as extra-virgin olive oil or flaxseed oil. If you must fry, *never allow the oil to smoke*— use a medium heat and use extra-virgin olive oil or a heat resistant oil such as cold-pressed peanut or sesame oil. For baking at temperatures above 350°F use butter.

○ Eat **cold water fish** such as mackerel, herring and salmon because they contain essential fatty acids for artery health.

○ **Fresh vegetable** and **fruit juices** are an excellent way to get minerals and detoxify your body. Fresh organic carrots, beets, parsley, apple, wheat grass and burdock root are excellent.

○ **Consume soy products** on a regular basis.

Herbal

● **Astragalus**—used when stimulation of the immune system is needed. Take 2 capsules or 60 drops three times daily.

● **Red clover**—historically used to detoxify the blood in cancer treatment. Take 30 drops twice daily. *Do not take if you are on blood thinning medications.*

○ **Shiitake mushroom**—this mushroom is commonly used in Japan as part of cancer treatment. It has the ability to stimulate the immune system to attack cancer cells. Take as directed on container.

○ **Licorice root** (12% glycyrrhizin)—stimulates the immune system. Take 1 capsule or 30 drops three times daily.

○ **Garlic**—used for both prevention and treatment of cancer by activating the immune system. Take 2 capsules or 30 drops three times daily.

○ **Onion**—used for both prevention and treatment of cancer by activating the immune system. Consume liberally.

○ **Burdock root**—detoxifies the liver and blood. Take 1 to 2 capsules or 30 to 60 drops three times daily.

○ **Reishi mushroom**—known for its ability to enhance immune system function. Take as directed on container.

○ **Echinacea** (4% echinacosides and 0.7% flavonoids)— enhances immune system activity. Take 2 capsules (250 mg each) or 60 drops three times daily.

○ **Milk thistle** (80% silymarin)—detoxifies the liver and body. Take 250 mg daily or 30 drops with each meal.

○ **Chlorophyll**—detoxifies the tissues. Take as directed on container.

○ **Blue-green algae**—detoxifies the tissues. Take as directed on container.

○ **Flaxseed oil**—supplies essential fatty acids for immune system health. Also contains lignans which have anti-carcinogenic properties. Take 1 to 2 tablespoons daily.

○ **Green tea**—contains potent antioxidants and may have anti-carcinogenic properties. Drink daily.

Vitamins and Minerals

● **High potency multi-vitamin without iron**—take daily.

● **Coenzyme Q10**—increases cell oxygenation and energy. As well, research is showing benefits for metastatic cancer. Take 150 to 300 mg daily.

● **Vitamin C with bioflavonoids**—stimulates the immune system. Take to the point where diarrhea starts and then cut back until stools are normal. Dosages can range from 1,000 to 20,000 mg daily.

○ **Beta-carotene**—stimulates the immune system and works as an antioxidant to protect the cells. Take a total of 100,000 to 200,000 IU daily.

○ **Vitamin E**—used for both prevention and treatment of cancer by activating the immune system. Take 400 to 800 IU daily.

○ **Zinc**—activates the immune system. Take 50 mg daily **with** 5 mg of **copper**.

○ **Selenium**—stimulates the immune system and works as an antioxidant to protect the cells. Take 200 mcg daily.

○ **B complex**—helps body with stress. Take 100 mg complex daily.

○ **Grape seed extract (PCO)**—stimulates the immune system. Take 100 to 150 mg daily.

Other

● **Shark cartilage**—stimulates the immune system and inhibits the growth of tumors. Typical dosage is 1 g for every two pounds of body weight.

- **Mental imagery** techniques are important to help activate the immune system and reduce stress. T'ai chi, yoga and daily exercise are excellent ways to alleviate stress.
- Consider **acupuncture** and **Chinese herbal medicine**
- O **Bovine cartilage**—very similar properties to shark cartilage. Take as directed on container.
- O **Thymus glandular**—stimulates the immune system. Take 1 tablet three times daily between meals.
- O **Counseling** helps the patient and family deal with the fear, grief and stress that comes with the diagnosis of cancer.
- O **Constitutional hydrotherapy**—see *Appendix A.*
- O Consider **homeopathy** from a qualified practitioner.

Canker Sores

Also referred to as apthous ulcers or stomatitis, canker sores are tiny ulcers that form on the inside lining of the mouth. These fluid-filled lesions can vary in size and are often painful. They have many causes and some of the most common ones I see are food allergies and sensitivities, nutritional deficiencies, flora imbalance and poor immune system resistance due to stress.

Nutrition

- **Avoid citrus fruit** (such as oranges, lemons, pineapple) and other **acidic foods** like tomatoes because they can aggravate or bring on this condition.
- O Identify and eliminate **food allergies** and **sensitivities** (see *Appendix E*). Wheat is a common allergen for this condition.
- O **Eat plain yogurt** as its bacteria can help heal these lesions.
- O **Avoid** spicy foods, alcohol, tobacco and refined sugar products because they can aggravate or bring on canker sores.

Herbal

- **Myrrh with goldenseal**—stimulates healing of the mouth tissue. Put 15 drops (or the contents of a capsule) of each in a small amount of water. Swish in mouth and swallow. Use three times daily until condition resolves.

○ **Licorice root** (12% glycyrrhizin)—heals irritated tissues. Take 1 capsule or 30 drops three times daily. Also available in tea form—use as a mouthwash three times daily.

○ **Peppermint tea**—soothes and promotes healing. Take 1 cup three times daily.

Vitamins and Minerals

○ **Zinc**—promotes healthy tissue growth. Take 30 mg daily with meals.

○ **Copper**—used with **zinc**. Take 3 mg daily with meals.

○ **High potency multi-vitamin without iron**—take daily to ensure against nutritional deficiencies.

○ **Vitamin C with bioflavonoids**—heals the mouth and gum tissues. Take 3,000 mg daily in divided doses.

○ **B complex**—excellent supplement to help the body deal with stress and known for its ability to prevent canker sores. Take a 50 mg complex daily.

Other

○ **Acidophilus**—helps balance the bacteria in the mouth. Take 2 capsules or 1/4 teaspoon three times daily.

○ **Homeopathic *Nat phos* 6x**—works as an acid/base balancer in system. Used to prevent and treat canker sores. Take a dose two to three times daily for treatment and prevention.

○ **Drink purified water only**.

Carpal Tunnel Syndrome

This syndrome is a complex of symptoms that occur when the median nerve (which runs through the wrist area) becomes compressed or swollen, usually due to repetitive use of the hands and wrists. Common symptoms include pain and weakness of the wrist and fingers. It has become much more wide-spread with the increased use of computers and is also common to musicians, athletes, restaurant workers, factory workers and many others who constantly use their hands and wrists. Pregnancy can also bring on carpal tunnel symptoms from the extra fluid in the wrist tissue.

Nutrition

○ **Avoid** the following because they increase inflammation: caffeine (coffee, tea, chocolate and soda pop), alcohol, tobacco products and refined sugars.

Herbal

● **Bromelain**—a natural anti-iflammatory. Take 500 mg three times daily between meals.

○ **Curcumin**—a natural anti-inflammatory. Take 250 mg three times daily between meals.

○ **Dandelion leaf**—useful for pregnant women that have a lot of water retention and swelling. Use under the supervision of a medical professional. Take 1 capsule or 30 drops three times daily.

Vitamins and Minerals

● **Vitamin B6**—a very important treatment because it reduces tissue swelling and inflammation of the affected nerves. Take 50 mg twice daily for a minimum of two months.

○ **B complex**—to enhance the effect of **vitamin B6** take a 50 mg complex daily.

○ **Calcium** and **magnesium**—to help with nerve healing take 1,000 mg daily of each with a meal.

Other

● **Homeopathic *Ruta* 30C**—indicated if there is a history of repetitive strain with the wrist. Take a dose two times daily.

● **Spinal manipulation** or **chiropractic** relieves pressure on the nerve.

● **Acupuncture** by a qualified practitioner.

○ **Proper biomechanics** are necessary to prevent carpal tunnel syndrome. Have a professional analyze your work area and make recommendations on a design specific for your body type and posture. For example, when typing, the wrists should be kept parallel to the floor.

○ Homeopathic *Kali phos* **6x** and *Mag phos* **6x**—heal the nerves. Take a dose of each three times daily.

○ **Massage** by a qualified practitioner.

○ **Physiotherapy** by a qualified practitioner.

Cataracts

This condition is characterized by a decrease in the transparency of the eye lens which results in a gradual loss of vision. The lens can be damaged by free radicals. Fortunately, the body uses certain vitamins called antioxidants to protect itself against this damage. Natural treatment seeks to decrease the amount of free radical damage while enhancing antioxidant status.

Nutrition

● Drink **juice** from fresh, organic vegetables and fruit for beta-carotene, antioxidants and enzymes. An excellent formula would contain carrots, beets and apples. Drink two to three glasses daily.

○ **Avoid** the following because they may accelerate cataract formation—dairy products, refined sugars, caffeine and alcohol.

○ Eat a diet high in **fruits, legumes** and **vegetables** for their mineral content.

Herbal

● **Cineraria**—historically used as an herbal treatment for cataracts. Use alone or as part of an herbal eye drop formula. Take as directed on container.

● **Bilberry** (25% anthocyanosides)—increases circulation to the eyes and is a strong antioxidant. Take 80 to 160 mg daily.

○ **Ginkgo** (24% standardized extract)—enhances circulation to the eyes and has an antioxidant effect within the eye tissue. Take 80 mg or 30 drops three times daily.

Look for formulas containing these herbs as well as eyebright and carrot juice powder.

Vitamins and Minerals

The following antioxidant vitamins protect the eye lens:
- **Vitamin C with bioflavonoids**—take 1,000 mg three times daily.
- **Beta-carotene**—take 100,000 IU daily.
- **Vitamin E**—take 800 IU daily.
- **Grape seed extract (PCO)**—take 50 mg three times daily.
- **Selenium**—take 400 mcg daily.
- ○ **Zinc**—take 30 mg daily **with** 3 mg of **copper**.
- ○ **High potency multi-vitamin without iron**—take daily with a meal to ensure against nutritional deficiencies.
- ○ **B complex**—take a 50 mg complex once daily.
- ○ **Vitamin A**—take a total of 25,000 IU daily.

Other

- **Acupuncture** or **Chinese herbal medicine** can be very effective.
- **Homeopathic eye drops**—natural healing for the eyes. Take as directed.
- ○ Wear **sunglasses** that protect against UV rays which accelerate cataract formation (see your optometrist).
- ○ If you have **diabetes** the blood sugar imbalance accelerates cataract formation (follow program under *Diabetes*).
- ○ **Homeopathic *Calc fluor* 6x**—natural healing for the eyes. Take a dose three times daily.

Cervical Dysplasia

This term refers to abnormal cells of the cervix (uterine opening). The Pap smear gives different gradings of abnormalities of the cells. A virus called the Human Papilloma Virus is believed to be the initiating cause of this condition. Cervical cancer can arise if the condition is not reversed in the early stages. Lifestyle and nutrition are an important part of the treatment program.

Nutrition

● It is advisable to follow a **plant-based diet** since red meat contains harmful saturated fat.

○ **Increase fiber**—add high fiber foods to the diet such as apples, oat bran, broccoli, Brussels sprouts, cabbage, carrots, wholegrain flour and green leafy vegetables.

○ **Increase water intake**—drink at least six to eight glasses of purified water daily.

○ **Avoid** refined sugar products, fatty foods, fried foods, margarine, alcohol, caffeine and dairy products.

○ Use **cold-pressed oils** such as extra-virgin olive oil or flaxseed oil. If you must fry, *never allow the oil to smoke*—use a medium heat and use extra-virgin olive oil or a heat resistant oil such as cold-pressed peanut or sesame oil. For baking at temperatures above 350°F use butter.

○ Eat **cold water fish** such as mackerel, herring and salmon because they contain essential fatty acids.

○ Eat **garlic, onions** and **legumes** liberally because they help detoxify the body.

Herbal

The following herbal formula is recommended for a minimum of three months:

● **Red clover**—purifies the blood. May have anti-carcinogenic properties. Take 1 capsule or 30 drops twice daily.

● **Dandelion root**—detoxifies the liver. Take 1 capsule or 30 drops twice daily.

● **Licorice root** (12% glycyrrhizin)—stimulates immune system and acts as a natural anti-inflammatory. Take 1 to 2 capsules or 30 to 60 drops twice daily.

● **Goldenseal**—stimulates the immune system and purifies the blood. Take 1 capsule or 30 drops twice daily.

Vitamins and Minerals

● **Folic acid**—this B vitamin is necessary for the proper division of the cervical cells. It is often deficient in women who are using or have used the birth control pill. Requirements also increase with pregnancy. Take 5 mg twice daily for three months, then cut back to 2.5 mg daily.

● **Beta-carotene**—protects DNA. Take 100,000 IU daily.

● **Vitamin A**—required for healthy replication of cervical cells. Take 10,000 IU daily with a meal.

○ **Vitamin C with bioflavonoids**—1,000 mg three times daily.

○ **Selenium**—antioxidant that protects DNA. Take 200 mcg daily.

○ **High potency multi-vitamin without iron**—take on a daily basis with meals to ensure against nutritional deficiencies.

Other

● Consider **homeopathy** from a qualified practitioner.

○ **Discontinue birth control pill** with the help of your doctor as it can promote or worsen this condition.

○ **Discontinue smoking** or avoid second-hand smoke.

○ **Constitutional hydrotherapy**—see *Appendix A*.

○ **Avoid unprotected intercourse**.

Cold

The common cold is caused by a variety of viruses that infect the upper respiratory system. Symptoms include fatigue, fever, headache and a runny nose. Best results are obtained when natural treatment is begun at the first appearance of a cold. One can reduce the length and severity of a cold with natural medicine even when treatment has begun midway through the illness.

Nutrition

○ **Eat lightly** because this conserves energy for the body by not having to use it for digestion. Eat foods such as home-made chicken soup.

○ **Drink plenty of fluids** such as purified water (six to eight glasses daily) and herbal tea.

○ **Avoid dairy and sugar** products because they can lower the immune system function.

Herbal

● **Echinacea** (4% echinacosides and 0.7% flavonoids)—stimulates the immune system and is antiviral. Take 2 capsules (250 mg each) or 60 drops every two hours until cold is gone.

● **Goldenseal**—stimulates the immune system and is antiviral. Take 2 capsules or 60 drops every two hours until cold is gone.

○ **Astragalus**—stimulates the immune system and is antiviral. Take 2 capsules or 60 drops every two hours until cold is gone.

○ **Garlic capsules**—stimulates the immune system and is antiviral. Take 2 capsules every two hours.

○ **Ginger tea**—promotes circulation in the body and alleviates pain. Especially effective if symptoms of fever, chills and nausea are present. Drink 1 cup every two hours.

○ **Yarrow tea**—especially helpful if fever is involved. Drink 1 cup every two hours.

Vitamins and Minerals

● **Vitamin C with bioflavonoids**—stimulates the immune system. Take 1,000 mg every two hours until cold is gone.

● **Zinc**—stimulates the immune system. Take 30 mg daily or suck on zinc lozenges, one every two hours.

○ **Beta-carotene**—maintains health of the respiratory tract lining. Take 100,000 IU daily until cold is gone.

○ **Multi-vitamin without iron**—taken on a daily basis can reduce the chance of catching a cold by supplying necessary nutrients to the immune system.

Other

● **Homeopathic cold formula**—take as directed on container for quick relief of symptoms.

● **Constitutional hydrotherapy**—see *Appendix A*.

- **Bed rest.**
- ○ **Foot hydrotherapy**—see *Appendix A*.

Cold Sores

These small blisters (also known as fever blisters) generally occur on the mouth and lips. They can also affect the genitals and eyes—see a medical professional in these cases. Cold sores are caused by the type 1 *herpes simplex* virus which remains dormant until an outbreak occurs. Their replication can be triggered by other infections (colds), sun and wind exposure, and stress (mental, physical and emotional).

Cold sores often begin with warning symptoms such as tingling and tenderness of the affected area. Over the course of a few days they turn from a small sore to a pus-filled blister. Natural medicine can be extremely effective in preventing and treating outbreaks.

Nutrition

- ○ If chronic cold sores are a problem you may have **food allergies** and **sensitivities** (see *Appendix E*).
- ○ Increase intake of **lysine** as it suppresses the growth of the virus. Foods with a high content of this amino acid include beans, eggs, brewer's yeast, potatoes and fish.
- ○ **Avoid arginine**, an amino acid that promotes the growth of the herpes virus. Foods with a high arginine content include chocolate, peanuts, other nuts, cereal grains, carob and raisins.

Herbal

- **Licorice root** (12% glycyrrhizin)—destroys the herpes virus. Take 2 capsules or 60 drops three times daily. This herb is also very effective as a **topical gel** application.
- ○ **Lomatium root**—stimulates the immune system and fights viruses. Take 2 capsules or 60 drops three times daily.

Vitamins and Minerals

- **Lysine**—an amino acid that stops the growth of the herpes virus. Take 1,000 mg daily between meals three times daily for acute episodes. Take 500 mg daily to prevent recurrences.
- ○ **Vitamin C with bioflavonoids**—stimulates the immune system. Take 1,000 mg three times daily.
- ○ **Vitamin E**—heals skin. Take 400 IU daily.
- ○ **Zinc**—stimulates the immune system. Take 30 mg daily.
- ○ **Copper**—works in conjunction with **zinc**. Take 3 mg daily.
- ○ **Selenium**—take 200 mcg daily to help prevent a recurrence.

Other

- **Homeopathic *Nat mur* 30C**—for acute symptoms take a dose every three hours for three days.
- **Homeopathic *Rhus tox* 30C**—for acute symptoms take a dose every three hours for three days.
- ○ **Ice**—when symptoms of an outbreak occur (i.e., tingling sensation) rub affected area with ice for five minutes every hour.
- ○ Consider **hypnosis** for chronic outbreaks.

Colic

A complex of symptoms that may include excessive crying, apparent abdominal pain and irritability. It usually occurs in infants between the ages of two to fourteen weeks. Different theories exist as to the cause of this condition such as disordered intestinal movement, imbalances in the nervous system, over- feeding, food allergies and intolerances, and family tension. The two most common causes I see are:

- breast-feeding stopped too early
- problems with the diet of the breast-feeding mother

Nutrition

- ○ Optimally the infant should be **breast-fed to at least six months of age**. Breast milk has all the nutrients necessary to mature the infant's digestive system quickly and properly.

○ Mothers that are breast-feeding should have a diet that **avoids the common triggers of colic**. These include dairy products, spicy foods, caffeine and brewer's yeast.

○ **Bottle formulas** that have a **soy base** should be used.

○ **Avoid** dairy-based bottle formulas.

Herbal

Herbs that decrease gas and spasm in the digestive tract.

● **Chamomile tea**—give 1/2 teaspoon of warm tea to infant every fifteen minutes for acute relief.

○ **Peppermint tea**—give 1/2 teaspoon of warm tea to infant every fifteen minutes for acute relief.

○ **Fennel tea**—give 1/2 teaspoon of warm tea to infant every fifteen minutes for acute relief.

Vitamins and Minerals

○ The mother should **discontinue vitamins** for two weeks to see if they are causing or aggravating the colic.

Other

● Consider **homeopathy** specific for your child from a qualified practitioner.

● **Homeopathic *Chamomile* 30C**—use as needed for effective relief of colic symptoms.

○ **Constitutional hydrotherapy** works well for infants. Use a face cloth to apply the treatment (see *Appendix A*).

○ **Homeopathic colic remedy**—as needed for relief of colic.

○ **Abdominal massage** moves the circulation and decreases spasm in the digestive tract. Use a combination of olive oil and peppermint oil. Massage the abdomen in a clockwise direction. Also massage the back. Perform once or twice daily.

○ Consider **chiropractic** or **laser acupuncture**.

Constipation

This term refers to the incomplete passage of feces or the need to strain in order to pass a bowel movement. From a naturopathic viewpoint, one should pass at least one fecal movement daily because efficient elimination prevents toxins from building up in the body.

Nutrition

- **Increase fiber**—a low fiber diet is the basis for chronic constipation. It is the weight of fiber that bulks up the stool to promote proper elimination. Add high fiber foods to the diet such as apples, oat bran, broccoli, Brussels sprouts, cabbage, carrots, wholegrain flour and green leafy vegetables.
- **Increase water intake**—drink at least six to eight glasses of purified water daily.
- Take a **fiber supplement** that has psyllium seed husks as the base of the formula. Take as directed on container. Drink at least eight ounces of water with each dose.
- ○ **Reduce intake of dairy products** as they can be constipating.
- ○ Identify and eliminate **food allergies** and **sensitivities** (see *Appendix E*).
- ○ **Unsweetened prune juice**—drink as needed (on a short-term basis only) to help move the bowels.

Herbal

- **Dandelion root**—stimulates digestion. Take 1 capsule or 30 drops with meals.
- ○ **Gentian root**—stimulates digestion. Take 1 capsule or 30 drops with meals.
- ○ **Ginger root**—stimulates digestion. Take 1 capsule or 30 drops with meals.
- ○ **Flaxseed oil**—take 1 tablespoon daily.

For acute relief, use the following herbs on a short-term basis. They are often used as a combination laxative formula.

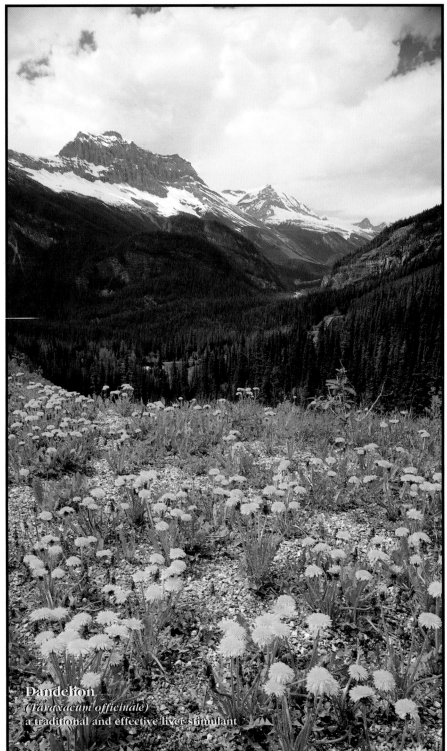

Dandelion
(Taraxacum officinale)
a traditional and effective liver stimulant

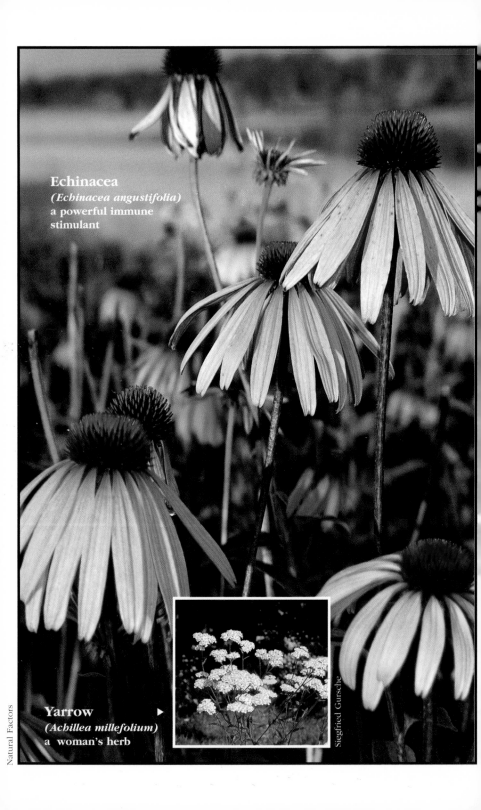

Echinacea
(Echinacea angustifolia)
a powerful immune
stimulant

Yarrow ▶
(Achillea millefolium)
a woman's herb

Siegfried Gursche

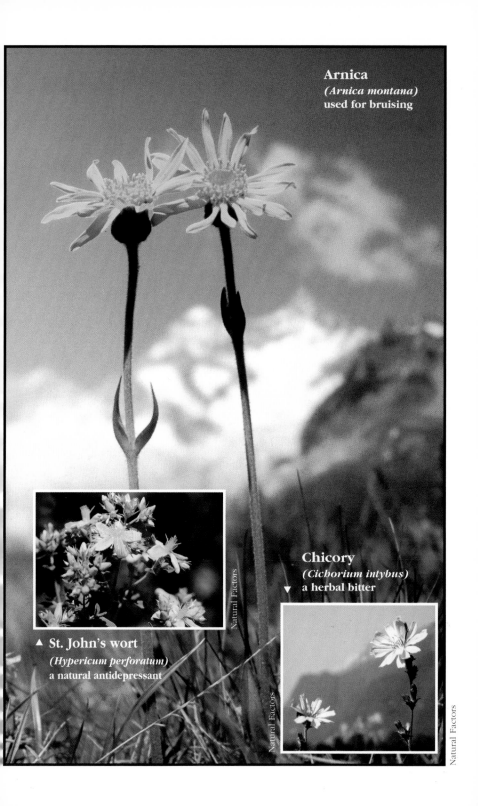

Arnica
(Arnica montana)
used for bruising

Chicory
(Cichorium intybus)
▼ a herbal bitter

▲ St. John's wort
(Hypericum perforatum)
a natural antidepressant

Natural Factors

Natural Factors

Natural Factors

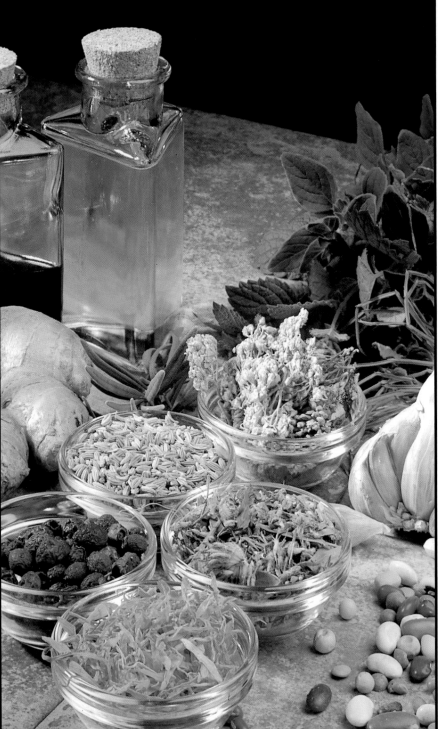

- **Cascara sagrada** (50% cascarosides)—take 1 capsule (200 to 250 mg) or 30 drops three times daily until the bowels are moving then stop using.
- **Senna** (4:1 leaf powder)—take 1 capsule (200 mg) or 30 drops three times daily until the bowels are moving then stop using.

Vitamins and Minerals

- **Vitamin C with bioflavonoids**—acts as a laxative at higher doses. Take 3,000 to 4,000 mg daily.
- **Magnesium**—acts as a laxative. Take 500 mg daily **as part of a calcium complex**. Use on a short-term basis.

Other

- **Go to the toilet each morning** upon awakening. This will help retrain the nervous system to eliminate consistently.
- **Exercise**—this is an underrated way to get the digestive organs functioning more optimally. Exercise three to five times weekly. Include exercises such as abdominal crunches to tone the muscles surrounding the colon.
- **Laxatives—avoid long-term use** of pharmaceutical or herbal laxatives as they make the colon lazy.
- **Caffeine** and **tobacco—reduce consumption** as they are stimulating and long-term use makes the colon lazy.
- Take time to **relax**—people who are uptight have a greater problem with constipation.

Cough

This reaction by the body occurs when the bronchial tubes become irritated from an environmental cause (such as dust) or infection. Mucus is produced by the body to help remove irritants. It is important to let the mucus be expelled continually while using the following therapies to be more comfortable and reduce the intensity and length of the cough.

Nutrition

○ **Avoid dairy** products—they are known to produce mucus. Use dairy alternatives such as soy cheese and rice milk.

○ **Avoid sugar** products because they lower immune function.

○ Chronic coughs may be related to **food allergies** and **sensitivities** (see *Appendix E*).

Herbal

● **Goldenseal**—immune stimulant, antibacterial and antiviral. Take 2 capsules or 60 drops every two hours.

● **Cherry bark**—a great herb for coughs. Take 2 capsules or 60 drops every two hours.

○ **Echinacea** (4% echinacosides and 0.7% flavonoids)—immune stimulant, antibacterial and antiviral. Take 2 capsules (250 mg each) or 60 drops every two hours.

○ **Tussilago**—soothes the respiratory passages and helps to expel mucus. Take 2 capsules or 60 drops every three hours. Do not use longer than one month.

○ **Mullein**—soothes an inflamed throat. Take 2 capsules or 60 drops every three hours.

○ **Garlic capsules**—immune stimulant, antiviral, antibacterial and good for coughs. Take 2 capsules three times daily or consume liberal amounts of garlic with meals.

Vitamins and Minerals

● **Vitamin C with bioflavonoids**—stimulates the immune system. Take 1,000 mg every three hours.

○ **Beta-carotene**—stimulates the immune system and is specific to the respiratory passages. Take 100,000 IU daily.

○ **Zinc**—stimulates the immune system. Take 50 mg daily until cough is gone.

Other

● **Constitutional hydrotherapy**—see *Appendix A*.

Cuts

Minor cuts can be treated effectively with natural medicine. Make sure to clean the wound thoroughly with soap and water to prevent infection. Use the following treatments to enhance skin healing.

Nutrition

○ **Avoid large amounts of sugar** products because they lower immune function.

Herbal

● **Calendula**—a superior herb tincture for disinfecting wounds as well as speeding up healing. Apply to cuts with a cotton ball three to four times daily.
○ **Comfrey**—apply cream to the cut three to four times daily.
○ **Cayenne pepper**—sprinkle on cut if bleeding is a problem (it helps stop minor bleeding).

Vitamins and Minerals

● **Vitamin E**—oil or gel applied topically after wound seals to prevent scar tissue. Apply twice daily for two weeks.
○ **Zinc**—promotes wound healing. Take 30 mg daily.
○ **Copper**—works in conjunction with **zinc**. Take 3 mg daily.
○ **Vitamin C with bioflavonoids**—promotes tissue healing. Take 1,000 mg three times daily.

Other

● **Homeopathic** *Calendula* **30C**—take a dose twice daily until cut is healed.

Dandruff

This condition occurs when large amounts of dead skin form flakes on the scalp. Overactive sebaceous glands are often involved in the formation of dandruff and nutritional deficiencies are a common underlying cause. Bacterial or fungal infections may also be present. Cradle cap is a similar condition found in infants.

Nutrition

○ **Avoid dairy** and **sugar** products.

○ Use **olive oil** as main source of oils in diet.

○ **Eat fatty fish** such as salmon, herring and mackerel for their essential fatty acid content.

○ **Review diet** of nursing mother for infant with cradle cap (see *Appendix E*).

Herbal

● **Flaxseed oil**—supplies essential fatty acids for skin health. Take 1 tablespoon or 3 capsules daily.

○ **Black currant oil**—supplies essential fatty acids for skin health. Take 1 tablespoon or 3 capsules daily.

○ **Burdock root**—detoxifies the skin. Take 1 capsule or 30 drops three times daily.

Vitamins and Minerals

● **B complex**—supplies necessary B vitamins for scalp health. Take a 50 mg tablet twice daily.

○ **Zinc**—for skin healing. Take 30 mg daily **with** 3 mg of **copper**.

○ **Biotin** and **vitamin B12**—talk to your physician about the use of these vitamins for treatment of cradle cap.

○ **High potency multi-vitamin without iron**—take daily to ensure against nutritional deficiencies.

○ **Vitamin C with bioflavonoids**—for optimal skin health take 1,000 mg three times daily.

Other

○ **Rub olive oil into scalp** each night as it provides essential fats for the scalp and prevents flaking.

○ Experiment with **different herbal shampoos** because certain shampoos can cause allergic reactions.

○ **Salmon oil**—supplies omega-3 fatty acids for skin health. Take 2 capsules (1,000 mg each) twice daily.

Depression

It is normal to experience feelings of depression for short periods of time. However, prolonged or unexplained depression should be examined and treated. Common symptoms of depression include fatigue, loss of interest in daily or pleasurable activities, sleep disturbance, feelings of worthlessness, mood swings, change in appetite and reduced ability to concentrate. Thoughts of suicide and death may be part of the picture.

Depression can have many causes and should be examined from a "whole person" perspective. Emotional feelings such as suppressed anger or unexpressed grief are commonly at the root of depression. As well, biochemical causes need to be examined. These include Seasonal Affective Disorder, food allergies and sensitivities, and hormone imbalances like hypothyroidism.

Nutrition

○ **Avoid** refined sugar products, artificial sweeteners, caffeine, alcohol and tobacco products.

○ Follow the **Elimination and Reintroduction Diet** (see *Appendix E*) to see if the depression improves.

Herbal

● **St. John's wort**—has been proven to be quite effective for mild to moderate depression, acting as a mood enhancer. Take 300 mg of standardized extract containing 0.3 percent hypericin two to three times daily.

● **Gotu kola**—improves mental function and mood. Take 1 capsule or 60 drops three times daily.

○ **Black cohosh**—a great herb for depression when one feels "like a black cloud is hanging over their head." Take 1 capsule or 30 drops of extract three times daily.

○ **Kava kava**—a relaxant and antidepressant. Take 1 capsule (100 mg) or 30 drops of extract twice daily.

Vitamins and Minerals

● **B complex**—many of the B vitamins are needed for the formation of neurotransmitters. Take a 50 mg complex once daily.

○ **L-Tryptophan**—an amino acid used to form the neurotransmitter serotonin which elevates mood. Take 2 g three times daily with a source of carbohydrates.

○ **Tyrosine**—another amino acid used to form necessary neurotransmitters for mood. Take 2 g three times daily.

○ **Vitamin B12**—a great vitamin for the nervous system. Talk to your physician about injections of B12.

Other

Imbalances of the following hormones can lead to depression:

○ **DHEA**—low levels of this hormone may be a contributing cause of depression. Have your levels tested by a physician. A typical adult dosage is 10 to 50 mg.

○ **Thyroid**—low thyroid function is quite common in women. Have your levels tested by a physician. Even when lab values are normal supplementation of thyroid glandular or Armour Thyroid may be helpful.

○ **Melatonin**—may be low and contribute to Seasonal Affective Disorder where people get depressed due to lack of sunshine. Supplementation of melatonin starting at 0.5 mg in the evening may help. As well, a better treatment may be the use of full spectrum lights (10,000 lux) for one hour daily.

● Consider **homeopathy** from a qualified practitioner.

○ **Counseling**—work with a qualified practitioner to find the cause of the depression.

○ **Exercise** is an underrated method of enhancing mood.

○ **Homeopathic *Kali phos* 6x** is a tonic for the nervous system. Take a dose three times daily.

○ **Pharmaceutical drugs**—review with your physician any

pharmaceutical drugs, including oral contraceptives, you are taking to see if depression is a side-effect.
○ Consider a form of **relaxation** like meditation or t'ai chi.

Diabetes

Diabetes mellitus is a condition where blood sugar levels can become greatly elevated. This can lead to serious complications such as atherosclerosis, kidney disease and nerve damage. There are two types of diabetes:

- **Insulin-dependent (type 1):** Associated with juvenile onset and insulin is required. Natural medicine serves to increase the health of the person with this condition. Insulin must continually be used.
- **Non-insulin-dependent (type 2):** Associated with adult onset and pharmaceutical drugs may, or may not, be needed depending on the severity. Natural medicine can often be a primary treatment in this type of diabetes.

Note: It is important that diabetics be closely monitored by a physician.

Nutrition

- **Increase fiber**—helps in regulating the absorption of glucose. Add high fiber foods to the diet such as apples, oat bran, broccoli, Brussels sprouts, cabbage, carrots, wholegrain flour and green leafy vegetables.
- Take a **fiber supplement** that has psyllium seed husks as the formula base. Drink eight ounces of water with each dose.
- Eat **cold water fish** such as salmon and mackerel as they contain essential fatty acids for blood sugar balance.
- **Food allergies** and **sensitivities** need to be identified as they promote blood sugar imbalance (see *Appendix E*).
- ○ Eat a diet high in **cereals, grains, vegetables, legumes** and other complex carbohydrates.
- ○ **Minimize** intake of all **simple sugars**.
- ○ **Increase water intake.**

○ **Brewer's yeast**—take 1 tablespoon twice daily for trace minerals and B vitamins necessary for blood sugar balance.

○ Eat **garlic** and **onions** frequently to balance blood sugar.

○ Eat **smaller, more frequent meals** throughout the day. Include protein sources throughout the day such as nuts, chicken and fish (unless kidney disease is involved).

Herbal

● *Gymnema sylvestre*—studies have shown it to have positive blood sugar balancing results. Take 400 mg of extract daily.

○ **Fenugreek**—balances blood sugar. Take capsules in an amount equivalent to 10 g daily with meals.

○ **Garlic**—stabilizes blood sugar. Consume liberally or take 1 capsule three times daily.

○ **Bilberry** (25% anthocyanosides)—this herb both balances blood sugar and protects the eyes and blood vessels with its antioxidants. Take 80 mg three times daily.

Vitamins and Minerals

The following vitamins and minerals are all useful supplements for diabetics. Given amounts should be the daily total, including a multi-vitamin.

● **Chromium**—helps to transport glucose into the cells. Take 400 mcg daily.

○ **B complex**—take a 100 mg complex once daily.

○ **Vitamin C with bioflavonoids**—take 1,000 mg four times daily.

○ **Vitamin E**—take 400 IU daily.

○ **Magnesium**—take 500 mg daily.

○ **Selenium**—take 200 mcg daily.

○ **Taurine**—take 500 mg twice daily.

○ **Zinc**—take 30 mg daily **with** 3 mg of **copper**.

Other

● Consider **homeopathy** from a qualified practitioner.

○ **DHEA**—may be a valuable hormone to prevent the progression of diabetes. Have levels checked by your physician. Common dosage is 25 to 100 mg daily.

○ **Glandular treatment**—the use of adrenal, pancreatic and thyroid glandulars help support the glands involved with blood sugar metabolism. Take a formula containing these glandulars (or take individually) three times daily between meals.

○ **Daily exercise** is important to help control blood sugar levels.

○ Consider **Chinese herbal medicine** from a qualified practitioner.

○ **Salmon oil**—supplies omega-3 fatty acids for artery and nerve health. Take 2 capsules (1,000 mg each) twice daily.

Diarrhea

This condition occurs when the body is attempting to rid itself of toxins or is dealing with an infection. Severe acute episodes or chronic diarrhea should be treated by a medical professional.

Nutrition

○ Eat **light meals** such as soups and stews.

○ Drink fluids composed of **dilute vegetable juices**.

○ Eat **bananas**.

○ Use **fluid replacement drinks** such as Recharge.

○ Use **pedialyte drink** for children to replace lost electrolytes.

○ Drink plenty of **purified water**.

○ Chronic bouts of diarrhea may be related to **food allergies** and **sensitivities** (see *Appendix E*).

Herbal

● **Slippery elm**—heals the lining of the digestive tract. Take 2 capsules or 60 drops four times daily.

● **Ginger**—reduces inflammation of the digestive tract. Take 2 capsules, 60 drops or 1 cup of tea four times daily.

○ **Goldenseal**—stimulates the immune system and is antiviral and antibacterial. Take 2 capsules or 60 drops four times daily.

○ **Marshmallow root**—soothes the lining of the digestive tract. Take 2 capsules or 60 drops four times daily.

Vitamins and Minerals

○ **Multi-vitamin**—take daily to help replace lost minerals. **Avoid extra** supplementation of **vitamin C and magnesium** as they may increase diarrhea.

Other

● **Charcoal capsules**—take 2 capsules of activated charcoal every three hours for acute diarrhea. Children over the age of five should take 1 capsule twice daily.
○ **Constitutional hydrotherapy**—see *Appendix A.*
○ **Homeopathic Combination Formula**—take as directed on container

Ear Infections

There are basically two types of middle ear infections:

• **Acute middle ear infection** (*otitis media*)—characterized by ear pain, irritability, fever and chills. It usually occurs in conjunction with a cold or upper respiratory tract infection.
• **Chronic middle ear infection** (*serous otitis media*)— characterized by chronic fluid in the inner ear, painless hearing loss and inability to equalize air pressure in the ears.

One major reason for the susceptibility in children is that the eustachian tube (the canal that drains fluid from middle ear and balances gas pressure) is horizontal and has a small diameter. As a child grows, this canal becomes more vertical and enlarges. Fluid is then able to drain properly whereas before it provided a breeding ground for bacteria. Children under the age of ten are the most susceptible to this condition. The other major cause is diet. Proper diagnosis by a physician should be made before treating these conditions.

Nutrition

- Infants that are fed breast milk have a lower incidence of ear infections. Optimally, **infants should be breast-fed for six months or longer.**
- **Children susceptible to ear infections should avoid** dairy products, citrus fruit, wheat products and sugar products as these are common causes of food sensitivities that promote this condition. Identify and eliminate **food allergies** and **sensitivities** (see *Appendix E*).
- ○ **Breast-feeding mothers** should **avoid dairy** products because they contain proteins which can depress immune system function.
- ○ **Bottle-fed infants** should be given a **soy-based formula** since it can be less allergenic than a cow's milk formula.
- ○ **Avoid** dairy-based bottle formulas.
- ○ **Eat** non-citrus fruits, dairy alternatives (such as rice milk, rice ice cream), beans, rice, wheat alternatives (such as quinoa, spelt, amaranth) and lots of vegetables.

Herbal

Note: Do not use drops if there has been any eardrum rupture.
- **Garlic oil drops**—put 3 warm drops in ear three times daily for acute infections.
- **Echinacea**—stimulates immune system and is antibacterial. Calculate the dosage for your child using *Appendix C*.
- ○ **Mullein drops**—put 3 warm drops in ear three times daily for acute infections.

Vitamins and Minerals

- **Vitamin C with bioflavonoids**—optimizes immune function. Dosage based on age times 500 mg per day.
- ○ **Beta-carotene**—optimizes immune function. Dosage based on age times 20,000 IU per day (100,000 IU maximum).
- ○ **Zinc**—optimizes immune function. Dosage based on age times 2.5 mg per day (15 mg maximum).

Other

- Children should **not be exposed to second hand smoke** as it increases risk of infections.
- Apply **alternating hot** (two minutes) and **cold** (30 seconds) **compresses** to affected ear. Repeat three times and perform every hour for acute episodes.
- **Homeopathic earache formula**—take a dose every two hours for two days.
- Consider **homeopathy** from a qualified practitioner if ear infections are a chronic problem.
- ○ **Bottle-fed infants** should be held in a **slightly upright position when feeding** to prevent fluid from blocking the eustachian tube.
- ○ **Constitutional hydrotherapy**—see *Appendix A.*
- ○ **Homeopathic** *Chamomile* **30C**—take a dose every hour for three doses and see if ear symptoms improve.
- ○ Consider **spinal manipulation** or **chiropractic** from a qualified practitioner.
- ○ **Constitutional** or **foot hydrotherapy**—see *Appendix A.*

Fatigue

This common complaint can have various causes and treatments. No underlying condition may be found but a medical professional should be consulted to rule out any disease process. The following natural therapies help to nourish the nervous and immune systems so that the body can increase its energy.

Nutrition

- ○ **Minimize caffeine consumption** because it decreases energy when used over an extended period of time.
- ○ **Minimize sugar consumption** as it lowers immune function.
- ○ **Rotate different grains** in the diet to optimize nutrition: amaranth, quinoa and spelt.

○ **Replace dairy products** with rice milk and soy milk products.

○ **Increase water intake**—drink at least six to eight glasses of purified water daily.

○ Identify and eliminate **food allergies** and **sensitivities** (see *Appendix E*).

Herbal

● **Siberian ginseng** (0.4% eleutherosides)—stimulates and nourishes the stress glands. Take 250 mg of a standardized extract or 30 drops two to three times daily.

● **Panax ginseng** (7% ginsenosides)—nourishes and regenerates the stress glands. Take 100 mg of a standardized extract two to three times daily.

○ **Milk thistle** (80% standardized silymarin)—improves liver function which indirectly increases energy levels. Take a daily total of 200 to 300 mg or 30 drops three times daily.

○ **Oatstraw**—builds up the nervous system. Take 1 capsule or 30 drops three times daily.

Vitamins and Minerals

● **Multi-vitamin without iron**—take one daily with a meal.

● **B complex**—involved with energy production. Take a 100 mg complex daily.

● **Vitamin B12**—have 1 mg injected by your physician twice weekly for four weeks, then once a week as needed.

○ **Vitamin C with bioflavonoids**—supports the stress glands. Take 1,000 mg three times daily.

○ **Magnesium**—take 250 mg twice daily.

○ **Coenzyme Q10**—take 90 mg daily with a meal.

Other

○ **Thyroid**—have your thyroid hormones tested by your physician as low levels can cause fatigue. Consider taking thyroid glandular at 1 tablet three times daily.

○ **DHEA**—this hormone is often low when chronic fatigue is a problem. Have your levels measured by your physician. An average adult dose is 10 to 50 mg.

○ Consider a form of **relaxation** like exercise, t'ai chi or a church group.

○ Consider **acupuncture** and **Chinese herbal medicine** from a qualified practitioner.

○ **Adrenal glandular**—stimulates and nourishes the adrenal glands. Take 1 tablet three times daily.

○ **Homeopathic *Kali phos* 6x**—nourishes the nervous system. Take a dose three times daily away from food or drink.

○ **Exercise**—a regular exercise program can help to build up energy over the long run.

○ **Blood tests**—performed by your doctor to rule out iron or vitamin B12 and folic acid deficiencies.

Fever

A fever is the body's attempt to stimulate the immune system to fight off foreign invaders such as bacteria and viruses. A temperature of 102 degrees is the optimal for the body to eliminate these and other organisms. Illness will be shortened when one works with the fever instead of suppressing (artificially lowering) it. Fevers of 104 degrees and higher may require medical attention.

Nutrition

● **Increase water intake**—drink six to eight glasses of purified water daily.

○ **Eat lightly if hungry, otherwise just drink fluids**: vegetable soups and broths are best.

○ **Avoid sugar and dairy** products because they can lower immune function.

Herbal

● **Echinacea** (4% echinacosides and 0.7% flavonoids)— stimulates the immune system. Take 2 capsules (250 mg each) or 60 drops every two to three hours.

● **Goldenseal**—stimulates the immune system. Take 2 capsules or 60 drops every two to three hours.

- **Yarrow**—promotes sweating and lowers fever. Take 1 cup of tea every two to three hours.
- ○ **Astragalus**—stimulates the immune system. Take 2 capsules or 30 drops every two to three hours.
- ○ **Ginger root**—stimulates circulation and wards off fever. Take 1 capsule, 30 drops or 1 cup of tea every two to three hours.
- ○ **Cinnamon tea**—stimulates circulation and wards off fever. Take 1 cup of tea every two hours.

Vitamins and Minerals

- ○ **Vitamin C with bioflavonoids**—stimulates the immune system. Take 1,000 mg every two hours.

Other

- **Homeopathic *Ferrum phos* 6x**—stimulates immune system. Take a dose every hour until fever decreases.
- **Constitutional hydrotherapy** is an excellent treatment for fever (see *Appendix A*).
- ○ **Foot hydrotherapy** works well for infants and children (see *Appendix A*).
- ○ **Bed rest**.
- ○ **Homeopathic fever formula**—stimulates the immune system. Take as directed on container.

Fibrocystic Breast Disease

This is not really a disease but a complex of symptoms. Fibrocystic refers to fluid-filled lumps in the breast that are usually painless and moveable during the month but which become tender the week prior to menstruation. Natural medicine works well to correct the underlying cause of fibrocystic breast disease. Common causes of this condition are dietary errors, hormonal imbalance and poor circulation.

Nutrition

- It is very important to **completely eliminate methylxan-**

thines from the diet. These are found in coffee, tea, chocolate and soda pop.

○ **Restrict** intake of **red meat**.

○ Eat large amounts of **fruit** and **vegetables**.

○ **Increase fiber**—add high fiber foods to the diet such as apples, oat bran, broccoli, Brussels sprouts, cabbage, carrots, wholegrain flour and green leafy vegetables.

○ Take a **fiber supplement** that has psyllium seed husks as the base of the formula. Take as directed on container. Drink at least eight ounces of purified water with each dose.

Herbal

The liver is responsible for breaking down hormones properly. Hormone imbalance may be involved with this condition.

The following herbs are used to tonify liver function:

● **Milk thistle** (80% silymarin)—take a daily total of 250 mg or 30 drops with each meal.

● **Phytolacca oil**—massaged on the breasts five times a week can be useful in reducing breast cysts.

● **Blessed thistle**—an excellent herb to prevent breast swelling and tenderness. Take 30 drops of extract twice daily.

○ **Dandelion root**—1 capsule or 30 drops with each meal.

○ **Burdock root**—1 capsule or 30 drops at the start of each meal.

The following oils are important because they provide essential fatty acids to reduce swelling:

● **Flaxseed oil**—take 1 tablespoon daily.

○ **Evening primrose oil**—take 3,000 mg daily.

Vitamins and Minerals

● **B complex**—Take a 50 mg complex once daily.

○ **Vitamin E**—has a long history of successful use in this condition. Take 800 IU daily for three months, then cut back to a maintenance dosage of 400 IU daily with meals.

Other

- **Natural progesterone cream**—can be extremely effective in helping to normalize hormonal balance. It is applied twice daily the last two weeks of the menstrual cycle and discontinued when the menstrual flow starts.
- ○ **Avoid using birth control pills** as they can promote or worsen this condition.
- ○ **Constitutional hydrotherapy**—see *Appendix A.*

Food Allergies and Sensitivities

Food allergies and sensitivities are an acquired problem. There are different degrees of reactions to various foods ranging from a runny nose or stomachache to a life threatening reaction like constriction of the throat. I find that food sensitivities improve when the source of the problem is addressed such as treating the digestion. When food is not broken down properly, larger than normal protein particles enter the bloodstream and are attacked by the immune system, creating physical symptoms. Also, it is common to become sensitive to foods one eats constantly. Variety in the diet will prevent this problem.

Nutrition

- ○ See *Appendix E* for **Elimination and Reintroduction Diet** to identify food sensitivities.
- ○ **Vary the foods in your diet**. See *Appendix D* for guidelines to a healthy diet.

Herbal

- **Plant enzymes**—help to break down food. Take with meals as directed on container.
- **Gentian root**—stimulates the digestive organs. Take 1 capsule or 30 drops with meals.

○ **Ginger root**—stimulates the digestive organs. Take 1 capsule or 30 drops with meals.

○ **Dandelion root**—stimulates the liver and gall-bladder to help digest fats. Take 1 capsule or 30 drops with meals.

Vitamins and Minerals

● **Quercitin**—helps allergies. Take 500 mg three times daily.

○ **Vitamin C with bioflavonoids**—works against allergies. Take 1,000 mg three times daily.

○ **B complex**—take a 50 mg complex daily.

Other

● Consider **homeopathy** by a qualified practitioner.

○ Follow a **juice fast** program to detoxify your system.

○ **Constitutional hydrotherapy**—improves digestion (see *Appendix A*).

○ Consider **acupuncture** and **Chinese herbal medicine**.

Fractures

Fractures are breaks or small cracks in the bone. The tissue surrounding the bone becomes swollen and contributes to the inflammation. A proper medical evaluation and setting of a fractured bone are necessary immediately after the injury. Afterwards natural medicine can be used to enhance the rebuilding and union of the bone.

Nutrition

○ **Avoid** foods and products that increase the excretion of calcium. These include caffeine, sugar, alcohol, tobacco, and salt.

○ **Avoid a high protein diet**.

○ Consume **whole grains** such as brown rice, oats, millet, barley, spelt, amaranth and quinoa.

○ Eat **soy rich foods**—they contain the chemicals dadzein and genistein that stop bone demineralization.

● The following foods are good **sources of calcium**:

Food Amount	Calcium Content
sardines 3 ounces	.375 mg
yogurt 1 cup (eight ounces)	.357 mg
collard greens 1 cup packed	.355 mg
whole milk 1 cup	.288 mg
sesame seeds 1/4 cup	.250 mg
turnip greens 1 cup	.250 mg
broccoli 1 cup	.180 mg
almonds 2 ounces	.150 mg
beans 1 cup	.150 mg
blackstrap molasses 1 tablespoon	.150 mg
kale 1 cup	.150 mg
salmon (canned) 3 ounces	.150 mg
tofu 4 ounces	.150 mg
apricots (dried) 1 cup	.100 mg

Herbal

○ **Comfrey**—stimulates bone healing. Applying a comfrey compress to the affected area on a daily basis is beneficial.

Vitamins and Minerals

● Many vitamins and minerals are known to be important in the prevention and reversal of bone loss. These include:

Supplement	Daily Amount
boron	.3 mg
copper	.3 mg
folic acid	.400–1,000 mcg
manganese	.10–20 mg
silicon	.1 mg
strontium	..5–3 mg
vitamin B6	.50 mg
vitamin C	.1,000 mg twice daily
vitamin D	.400 IU
vitamin K	.200–400 mcg
zinc	.30 mg

- **Calcium**—an integral component for bone formation. Take 500 mg twice daily with meals.
- **Magnesium**—essential for bone formation. Take 500 mg twice daily with meals.

Other

- **Homeopathic *Symphytum* 30C**—specific for healing broken bones. Take a dose twice daily for two to four weeks.
- ○ **Homeopathic *Calc phos* 6x**—specific for the union of bones. Take a dose twice daily until fracture is healed.
- ○ Consider **acupuncture** from a qualified practitioner to help with the pain and stimulate bone healing.

Gallstones

Bile, which is produced in the liver and stored in the gall-bladder, is used to digest fats. When needed, bile is released into the small intestine where the process of fat digestion begins. Gallstones block the opening to the gall-bladder resulting in symptoms such as bloating, gas and nausea after a fatty meal. Intense abdominal pain can also be experienced. There are different types of gallstones but the most common ones are saturated with cholesterol. This condition is mainly related to diet. It is easier to prevent gallstones but once they have formed it is important to reduce the susceptibility to flare-ups.

Nutrition

- Follow the **Elimination and Reintroduction Diet** (see *Appendix E*) to identify any foods that may trigger gall-bladder symptoms.
- ○ **Eat** a diet that is low in fat, sugar, caffeine and alcohol.
- ○ Take a **fiber supplement** that has psyllium seed husks as the base of the formula. Take as directed on the container. Drink at least eight ounces of purified water with each dose.
- ○ **Eat foods that detoxify the liver** such as beets, radish, carrots, artichokes, watercress and parsnips.

○ **Avoid rapid weight loss** programs as they can cause a predisposition to gallstones.
○ Drink six to eight glasses of **purified water** daily.

Herbal

● **Milk thistle** (80% silymarin)—helps with bile production and liver and gall-bladder detoxification. Take 250 mg or 30 drops with each meal.
● **Artichoke**—helps reduce blood lipids and gall-bladder inflammation. Take 1 capsule or 30 drops daily with meals for two months.
○ **Dandelion root**—helps bile production. Take 1 capsule or 30 drops daily with meals for two months.
○ **Tumeric extract**—take 50 to 100 mg with each meal.
○ *Dioscorea*—can be used short-term for gall-bladder pain. Take 1 capsule or 30 drops four times daily until symptoms resolve.

Vitamins and Minerals

The following supplements work to balance cholesterol saturation in the bile:
● **Choline**—take 1 g daily with a meal.
○ **Lecithin**—take 4 g daily with a meal.
○ **L-Methionine**—take 1 g daily with a meal.
○ **Taurine**—take 1,000 mg daily.
○ **Vitamin C with bioflavonoids**—take 1,000 mg daily.

Other

● Consider **acupuncture** and **Chinese herbal medicine** from a qualified practitioner.
○ **Constitutional hydrotherapy**—see *Appendix A*.

Gout

This condition arises when uric acid, a product of protein metabolism, accumulates in joint tissue. As a result, arthritic pain and swelling occurs. The classic area affected is the big toe. Diet, digestion and weight control are key areas that need to be addressed for improvement of this condition.

Nutrition

- **Avoid foods with a high purine content** because it is converted into uric acid. These include meats, shellfish, sardines, mackerel, herring and anchovies. Limit the intake of poultry, fish and legumes in general.
- Eat plenty of **fresh cherries** and **blueberries** because they reduce uric acid levels.
- ○ **Alcohol must be avoided** as it accelerates the formation of uric acid.
- ○ Drink six to eight glasses of **purified water** daily.
- ○ **Avoid** the following because they increase inflammation: caffeine (coffee, tea, soda pop), alcohol, tobacco and sugar.

Herbal

The following herbs help to promote proper protein digestion:
- **Plant enzymes**—help to metabolize food properly. Take as directed on container with meals.
- ○ **Dandelion root**—stimulates the gall-bladder to produce bile. Take 1 capsule or 30 drops daily with each meal. As well, it helps to detoxify the liver and the joints.

Other useful herbs:
- *Urtica urens*—for treatment of gout. Take 30 drops twice daily.
- ○ **Devil's claw**—useful during acute attacks of gout because it is a natural anti-inflammatory and may reduce uric acid levels. Take 2 capsules or 60 drops three times daily.
- ○ **Bromelain**—a natural anti-inflammatory. Take 500 mg three times daily between meals.

Vitamins and Minerals

- **B complex**—includes many B vitamins involved in protein metabolism. Take a 50 mg complex twice daily.

○ **Folic acid**—has been shown to reduce uric acid levels. Take a daily total of 20 mg.

○ **Vitamin C with bioflavonoids**—helps to mobilize uric acid from the tissues and excrete it from the body. Take 3,000 mg daily in divided doses.

Other

● Consider a three to five day **juice fast** to detoxify the body and joint tissues.

● **Homeopathic** *Colchicum* **30C**—useful for acute flare-ups of gout. Take a dose twice daily until acute symptoms resolve.

○ Consider specific **homeopathy** from a qualified practitioner.

○ **Homeopathic** *Nat phos* **6x**—used as an acid balancer. Take a dose three times daily.

○ **Weight loss**—takes stress off the joints as well as reducing uric acid levels.

○ **Constitutional hydrotherapy**—see *Appendix A.*

Gum Disease (Gingivitis)

This is a condition of swelling and inflammation of the gums. It is the beginning stage of periodontal disease (disease of the gums, teeth and surrounding structures). Nutritional and hygienic treatment are needed to improve this condition.

Nutrition

○ Eat **leafy green vegetables** for mineral and vitamin content.

○ **Avoid sugar** products because they can promote bacterial growth and cavities.

○ Eat fruit such as **blueberries** and **grapes** as they contain substances that strengthen the gum tissue.

Herbal

● **Myrrh** and **goldenseal rinse**—mix myrrh (15 drops or 1/2 capsule) and goldenseal (15 drops or 1/2 capsule) in a small cup of warm water. Swish in mouth and swallow. Use this mixture twice daily.

Vitamins and Minerals

● **Vitamin C with bioflavonoids**—strengthens the gum tissue. Take 1,000 mg three times daily.

● **Folic acid**—decreases inflammation of the gums. Rinse mouth and swallow with a 0.1% solution twice daily.

○ **Grape seed extract (PCO)**—strengthens the gum tissue. Take 50 mg three times daily.

○ **Coenzyme Q10**—strengthens gum tissue. Take 100 mg daily.

○ **Vitamin E**—a natural anti-inflammatory that promotes tissue health. Take 400 IU daily.

○ **High potency multi-vitamin without iron**—take daily to ensure against nutritional deficiencies.

Other

● **Homeopathic *Calc fluor* 6x**—excellent medicine to heal gum tissue. Take a dose three times daily.

● **Avoid use of tobacco**—both smoking or chewing.

○ **Mercury filling removal**—chronic cases of gingivitis may improve with the proper removal of mercury fillings.

○ **Floss and brush teeth after meals**. Use a soft bristled toothbrush so the gums are not irritated.

Headache

There are various types of headaches, each with its own cause. Two of the more common ones are:

• **Tension headaches**—occur when stress causes tightening of the muscles which interferes with blood flow to the head region. The pain commonly extends from the shoulders and neck into the back of the head.

• **Migraine headaches**—are often on one side of the head with severe throbbing or aching. It may be preceded by nausea or a change in vision. This type of headache is more related to what is going on inside the body. Common causes include hormone imbalance, inefficient digestion (leads to increased toxins in the body), sluggish liver (the liver breaks down toxins in the body) and food sensitivities.

Nutrition

● **Avoid the following** (known to cause or aggravate headaches, especially migraines) for a period of three weeks to see if there is a reduction in the frequency and intensity of headaches: caffeine products, alcohol, tobacco, sugar, chocolate, dairy products, wine (red and white), and MSG and other preservatives.
● Identify and eliminate **food sensitivities** (see *Appendix E*).
○ Eat **non-packaged food:** fruits, vegetables and other un-processed foods.

Herbal

For hormonal balance:
○ **Vitex**—take 1 capsule or 30 drops twice daily.
○ *Dioscorea*—women should take 1 capsule or 30 drops three times daily for the last fourteen days of cycle.

For improved digestion:
● **Gentian root**—take 1 capsule or 30 drops at beginning of each meal.
○ **Ginger root**—take 1 capsule or 30 drops at beginning of each meal.
○ **Plant enzymes**—take as directed on container with meals.

For improved liver function:
○ **Milk thistle** (80% silymarin)—250 mg or 30 drops with each meal.
○ **Dandelion root**—take 1 capsule or 30 drops at each meal.
○ **Burdock root**—take 1 capsule or 30 drops at each meal.

For muscle relaxation:
○ **Valerian**—take 300 mg capsule or 30 drops two to three times daily.

For general prevention of headache:
○ **Feverfew** (0.2% parthenolides)—long history of successful use in preventing headaches. Take 250 mg or 30 drops three times daily.

Vitamins and Minerals

● **B complex**—aids body in dealing with stress at a biochemical level. Take a 50 mg complex once daily.
○ **Calcium and magnesium**—relaxes the nervous system and muscles. Take 500 mg of each in the evening with dinner.

Other

● For **acute headache** see *Appendix A* for directions on **foot hydrotherapy**.
● Consider **acupuncture** from a qualified practitioner for all types of headaches.
○ **Exercise**—relieves muscular, mental and emotional tension.
○ **Homeopathic Kali phos** **6x**—nourishes the nervous system. Take a dose three times daily.
○ Consider **spinal manipulation** or **chiropractic** from a qualified practitioner for tension headaches.
○ Consider **massage therapy** from a qualified practitioner for tension headaches.
○ Consider **homeopathy** from a qualified practitioner.

Heartburn

This condition occurs when acid from the stomach refluxes into the throat, usually after eating. A burning sensation is felt in the upper chest and can extend to the throat. The key to natural treatment of heartburn is to remove foods that upset the stomach, as well as to improve digestion.

Nutrition

- The following are known to aggravate heartburn so **minimize intake** of them: coffee, alcohol, milk, spicy foods, orange juice and tobacco.
○ Identify and eliminate **food sensitivities** (see *Appendix E*).
○ Drink **fresh fruit** and **vegetable juices**.
○ Eat **smaller, more frequent meals.**
○ Drink six to eight glasses of **purified water** daily.

Herbal

The following herbs are all soothing to the digestive system:
- **Slippery elm**—take 1 capsule or 30 drops with meals.
○ **Chamomile tea**—drink 1 cup with every meal.
○ **Peppermint tea**—drink 1 cup with every meal.
○ **Deglycyrrhizinated licorice root**—take 1 to 2 chewable tablets three times daily on an empty stomach.

Vitamins and Minerals

○ **Calcium**—natural antacid. Take 1,000 mg with evening meal.

Other

○ **Exercise**—exercising will help to prevent heartburn.
○ **Homeopathic *Nat phos* 6x**—works as an acid/base balancer. Take a dose three times daily away from meals.

Heart Disease

Heart disease can include many conditions that affect the heart such as congestive heart failure, cardiomyopathy and mitral valve prolapse. There are a variety of natural treatments that have beneficial effects. Contributing factors to this condition include atherosclerosis, high blood pressure, nutritional deficiencies and stress. It is these factors that need to be addressed in order to treat the cause of this serious condition.

Nutrition

- It is advisable to follow a **plant-based diet** since red meat contains harmful saturated fat.
- ○ **Dramatically increase intake of fruit and vegetables**.
- ○ **Increase fiber**—add high fiber foods to the diet such as apples, oat bran, broccoli, Brussels sprouts, cabbage, carrots, wholegrain flour and green leafy vegetables.
- ○ **Water soluble fiber**—increase intake of oat bran, pectin containing foods such as apples, and rice bran as they lower cholesterol.
- ○ Take a **fiber supplement** that has psyllium seed husks as the base of the formula. Take as directed on container. Drink at least eight ounces of purified water with each dose.
- ○ **Increase water intake**—drink at least six to eight glasses of purified water daily.
- ○ **Drink purified water** and **avoid chlorine-containing water** as it can promote atherosclerosis.
- ○ **Avoid** refined sugar products, fatty foods, fried foods, margarine and dairy products.
- ○ Use **cold-pressed oils** such as extra-virgin olive oil or flaxseed oil. If you must fry, *never allow the oil to smoke*—use a medium heat and use extra-virgin olive oil or a heat resistant oil such as cold-pressed peanut or sesame oil. For baking at temperatures above 350°F use butter.
- ○ Eat **cold water fish** such as mackerel, herring and salmon because they contain essential fatty acids for artery health.
- ○ Eat **garlic, onions** and **legumes** liberally because they help detoxify the arteries.
- ○ **Avoid** caffeine, alcohol and tobacco products.
- ○ **Limit sodium intake** to less than 3 g daily.

Herbal

- **Hawthorn**—increases blood flow in the vessels leading to the heart. Take a 250 mg capsule or 30 drops three times daily.
- **Garlic**—improves circulation as well as reduces cholesterol and fats in the blood. Take 4,000 mcg standardized allicin extract daily and consume garlic liberally.

○ **Ginkgo** (24% standardized extract)—improves circulation throughout the cardiovascular system. Take 60 mg three times daily.

○ **Bromelain**—breaks down plaques in the blood vessels. Take 500 mg three times daily between meals.

Vitamins and Minerals

● **Coenzyme Q10**—a nutrient needed for efficient heart contraction. Take 80 mg two to three times daily.

● **Magnesium**—used by the body to dilate blood vessels (including arteries to heart). Take 500 mg daily.

○ **L-Carnitine**—used by the heart muscle to efficiently utilize fatty acids for energy. Take 500 mg three times daily.

○ **B complex**—supplies a complex of vitamins for energy and stress glands. Take a 50 mg complex once daily.

○ **Vitamin C with bioflavonoids**—strengthens blood vessel walls. Take 3,000 mg daily in divided doses.

○ **Grape seed extract (PCO)**—strengthens the blood vessels. Take 50 mg twice daily.

Other

● Consider **chelation therapy** from a qualified practitioner.

● Consider **acupuncture** and **Chinese herbal medicine** from a qualified practitioner.

○ **Constitutional hydrotherapy**—promotes circulation through the cardiovascular system (see *Appendix A*).

○ **Stress relaxation** techniques—exercise, yoga, t'ai chi and mental imagery.

○ **Salmon oil**—supplies omega-3 fatty acids for artery health. Take 2 capsules (1,000 mg each) two to three times daily.

Hemorrhoids

This condition involves the swelling of the veins and supporting tissues of the rectum and anus. Symptoms include rectal pain, itching, bleeding and burning. Diet, lack of exercise and pregnancy are the most common causes of hemorrhoids.

Nutrition

- A **high fiber diet** is the most important nutritional concern. This helps reduce and prevent constipation and straining with bowel movements due to constipation. This lessens pressure on the veins in the rectal area so that they become less swollen. Include **fruit, vegetables, legumes** and **grains** as a large part of the diet.
- **Avoid** foods known to irritate hemorrhoids such as tomatoes, peanuts, caffeine, soda pop, spicy foods and citrus fruit.
- ○ Take a **fiber supplement** that has psyllium seed husks as the base of the formula. Take as directed on container. Drink at least eight ounces of purified water with each dose.
- ○ Identify and eliminate **food allergies** and **sensitivities** as they can aggravate hemorrhoids (see *Appendix E*).
- ○ **Eat a diet low in red meat.**

Herbal

The following herbs shrink hemorrhoid tissue:
- **Collinsonia root**—2 capsules or 30 drops three times daily.
- ○ **Horse chestnut**—2 capsules or 30 drops three times daily.
- ○ **Butcher's broom** (10% ruscogenin)—take 300 mg or 30 drops three times daily.

Vitamins and Minerals

The following vitamins help heal hemorrhoids:
- **Vitamin C with bioflavonoids**—take 1,000 mg three times daily.
- ○ **Grape seed extract (PCO)**—take 1 capsule (50 mg) three times daily.
- ○ **Vitamin E**—take 400 IU once daily with meals.

Other

- **Exercise**—helps to tone the blood vessels. Engage in aerobic exercise at least three times weekly.

- **Alternating sitz baths**—enhances circulation and remove congestion from swollen tissue. Sit in a large container of hot water for 3 minutes. Then get out and sit in a container of slightly cool water for 30 seconds. Repeat this alternation three times. Perform daily until condition resolves.
- **Constitutional hydrotherapy**—see *Appendix A*.
- **Homeopathic *Calc fluor* 6x**—take a dose three times daily. Also useful in preventing hemorrhoids.
- Consider **Chinese herbal medicine** from a qualified practitioner.

High Blood Pressure (Hypertension)

This is a common health problem related to diet and lifestyle factors. A "normal" reading for blood pressure is close to 120/80. If you have high blood pressure, regular check-ups with your physician are essential. Diet, lifestyle and herbal medicine are effective natural treatments for this condition.

Nutrition

- **Minimize** intake of fatty foods, alcohol, refined sugars and salt. Limit sodium intake to less than 3 mg daily.
- **Consume foods that are high in potassium** such as green vegetables, whole wheat, bananas, grapes, peaches, plums, pumpkin, squash, potatoes, beets, brewer's yeast and zucchini.
- **Whole foods** should be eaten with an emphasis on **vegetables** and **fruits**. Fruits and vegetables that are **freshly juiced** are excellent.
- **Garlic** and **onions** should be eaten liberally.
- Eaten on a regular basis, **celery** is helpful as it promotes the excretion of excess fluids and decreases blood pressure.
- **Increase fiber**—add high fiber foods to the diet such as apples, oat bran, broccoli, cabbage, carrots, wholegrain flour, psyllium husks and green leafy vegetables.

○ **Increase water intake**—drink at least six to eight glasses of purified water daily.

○ Identify and eliminate **food allergies** and **sensitivities** as they can aggravate hypertension (see *Appendix E*).

Herbal

● **Garlic**—improves circulation as well as reducing cholesterol and fats in the blood. Take 4,000 mcg standardized allicin extract three times daily.

○ **Hawthorn berry**—lowers blood pressure and improves heart contractions. Take a 250 mg capsule or 30 drops three times daily.

○ **Ginkgo** (24% standardized extract)—improves circulation throughout the cardiovascular system.

○ **Flaxseed oil**—contains essential fatty acids which help in lowering blood pressure. Take 2 tablespoons daily.

○ **Dandelion leaf** (4:1 extract)—acts as a mild diuretic so that excess fluids are excreted. Take 1 capsule (125 mg) or 30 drops three times daily.

Other useful herbs that have a diuretic action to lower blood pressure include uva ursi, juniper berry, cranberry and parsley.

Vitamins and Minerals

○ **Calcium**—has been shown to be valuable for this condition. Take 500 mg twice daily with a meal.

○ **Magnesium**—has a relaxing effect on the blood vessels. Take 500 twice mg daily with a meal.

○ **Coenzyme Q10**—lowers blood pressure when taken over a long term. Take 60 mg three times daily.

○ **Vitamin C with bioflavonoids**—may be beneficial in lowering blood pressure. Take 1,000 mg three times daily.

○ **Potassium**—if the diet is not high in fruit and vegetables take 300 to 600 mg daily.

Other

○ **Exercise**—it is crucial to follow a regular exercise program.

○ **Stress reduction** techniques—counseling, mental imagery and biofeedback are all useful.

○ Consider **acupuncture** from a qualified practitioner.

○ Consider **chelation therapy**—it is designed to bind then excrete toxic heavy metals such as cadmium which have been linked to high blood pressure.

HIV (AIDS)

HIV (Human Immunodeficiency Virus) is the virus that may result in AIDS (Acquired Immunodeficiency Syndrome). Persons with AIDS develop immune system breakdown resulting in a greater risk of infections and other illnesses. It should be noted that not all persons with HIV have AIDS. There are certain clinical criteria for one to be diagnosed with AIDS. Transmission of HIV occurs through HIV infected body fluids. There is no cure for AIDS. Natural medicine is under intensive research for its contribution to the treatment of HIV-positive individuals and those infected with AIDS.

Nutrition

○ It is advisable to follow a **plant-based diet** since red meat contains harmful saturated fat. The **intake of fruits and vegetables should be dramatically increased.**

○ **Increase fiber**—add high fiber foods to the diet such as apples, oat bran, broccoli, Brussels sprouts, cabbage, carrots, wholegrain flour and green leafy vegetables.

○ **Increase water intake**—drink at least six to eight glasses of purified water daily.

○ Avoid refined sugar products, fatty foods, fried foods, margarine and dairy products.

○ Use **cold-pressed oils** such as extra-virgin olive oil or flaxseed oil. If you must fry, *never allow the oil to smoke*— use a medium heat and use extra-virgin olive oil or a heat resistant oil such as cold-pressed peanut or sesame oil. For baking at temperatures above 350°F use butter.

○ Eat **cold water fish** such as mackerel, herring and salmon because they contain essential fatty acids for artery health.

○ Eat **garlic, onions** and **legumes** liberally because they help detoxify the arteries.

○ **Avoid** caffeine, alcohol and tobacco products because they produce toxins.

Herbal

The following herbs have antiviral properties:

● **Astragalus**—take 1 capsule or 30 drops three times daily.

● **Hypericum** (0.125% extract)—inhibits retroviruses like HIV. Take 300 mg or 30 drops of extract three times daily.

○ **St. John's wort** (0.3% hypericin)—currently being studied for its benefit against HIV. Take 300 mg capsule or 30 drops three times daily.

○ **Echinacea** (4% echinacosides and 0.7% flavonoids)—take 250 mg or 30 drops three times daily for short-term secondary infections.

○ **Reishi mushroom**—known for its ability to enhance the immune system. Take as directed on container.

Vitamins and Minerals

● **High potency multi-vitamin**—take daily to ensure against nutritional deficiencies.

○ **Coenzyme Q10**—an antioxidant that protects cells from damage. Take a total of 160 mg daily.

○ **Zinc**—needed for proper immune function. Take a daily total of 50 mg **with** 6 mg of **copper**.

○ **B complex**—helps the body deal with stress. Take a 100 mg complex once daily.

○ **Vitamin C with bioflavonoids**—stimulates the immune system. Take up to the point where diarrhea starts and then cut back until stools are normal. Dosages can range from 3,000 to 20,000 mg daily.

Other

- **Mental imagery** techniques are important to help activate immune system and reduce stress. T'ai chi, yoga and daily exercise are excellent ways to alleviate stress.
- Consider **acupuncture** and **Chinese herbal medicine** from a qualified practitioner.
- ○ **Counseling** helps patients and families deal with the fear, grief and stress that comes with the diagnosis of HIV.
- ○ **Constitutional hydrotherapy**—see *Appendix A*.
- ○ Consider **homeopathy** from a qualified practitioner.

Hyperactivity (ADHD)

Hyperactivity is now known as Attention Deficit Hyperactivity Disorder (ADHD). It refers mainly to children who experience problems with learning and behavior. My experience is that nutritional therapy and homeopathy offer the best fundamental treatment of this condition.

Nutrition

- **Identify** and **eliminate** food sensitivities—see *Appendix E*.
- ○ **Avoid all foods that contain preservatives**. Fresh whole foods should be eaten whenever possible.
- ○ **Avoid sugar**.

Herbal

- ○ **Passion flower**—a calming herb for the nervous system. A forty pound child can be given 15 drops of this herb three times daily. See *Appendix C* to calculate child's dosage.
- ○ **Flaxseed oil**—supplies essential fatty acids for proper nervous system formation. Children ages two to four can take half a tablespoon daily and children over four years of age can take 1 tablespoon daily.
- ○ **Gotu kola**—improves concentration. A forty pound child can be given 15 drops three times daily. Adult dosage is 1 to 2 capsules or 30 drops three times daily.

○ **Ginkgo** (24% standardized extract)—improves memory and concentration. A forty pound child can take 60 mg twice daily or 15 drops three times daily. Adult dosage is 60 mg or 30 drops three times daily.

Vitamins and Minerals

○ **Children's multi-vitamin** (without preservatives or dyes)— take one daily.

○ **Calcium and magnesium**—nourish and relax the nervous system. I recommend 500 mg daily of each with a meal (*for children two years of age and older*).

○ **Vitamin B6**—may be useful at higher doses for this condition. Take 50 to 100 mg daily (take under supervision).

○ **Grape seed extract (PCO)**—works against allergies. Take 50 mg daily.

Other

● **Homeopathy**—the most effective treatment I have seen for this condition. It is important to see a qualified practitioner for individualized treatment. An excellent book on this topic is *Ritalin Free Kids* by Doctors Ullman and Reichenberg-Ullman (Prima Publishing).

○ **Aluminum or lead toxicity**—these heavy metals have been shown to cause behavioral problems. Your physician should rule this out by having lab tests done.

○ **Homeopathic *Kali phos* 6x** and ***Mag phos* 6x**—nourish and relax the nervous system. Take a dose of each three times daily away from meals.

○ **Counseling**—involving the child and family to address any possible underlying emotional causes of the behavior.

Hypothyroid

The thyroid gland has a regulating effect on cell metabolism. When it is functioning below optimal level symptoms such as dry skin, constipation, cold hands and feet, depression, menstrual irregularities and weight gain can occur. This condition is more common in women and is often overlooked. Diagnosis is based on symptoms and lab results.

Nutrition

○ The thyroid gland needs **iodine** to make hormones. **Raw foods** that interfere with this process and **that should be avoided** include: cabbage, mustard, soybean, peanuts, turnips and millet. Cooking these foods will deactivate their harmful actions.

○ **Seafoods** like lobster, clam, kelp, oysters and sardines are healthy for the thyroid.

Herbal

○ **Kelp**—contains an organic form of iodine. Take as directed on container.

Vitamins and Minerals

The following vitamins are used to manufacture thyroid hormone.

○ **Zinc**—take 30 mg daily.

○ **Copper**—take 3 to 5 mg daily.

○ **Vitamin A**—take 25,000 IU daily.

○ **Vitamin C with bioflavonoids**—take 1,000 mg daily.

○ **B complex**—take a 50 mg complex once daily.

Other

● Consider **homeopathy** from a qualified practitioner.

○ **Adrenal glandular**—nourishes the stress glands which help support the thyroid gland. Take 1 tablet three times daily between meals. Should be taken for at least one month.

○ **Pituitary glandular**—supports the pituitary gland which is involved in stimulating thyroid hormone production. Take 1 tablet three times daily between meals. Should be taken for at least one month.

○ **Thyroid glandular**—stimulates thyroid production naturally. Take 1 tablet three times daily between meals. It should be taken for at least one month.

○ **DHEA**—replenishes stress hormones which support the thyroid gland. Take 20 to 50 mg daily under the supervision of a physician.

○ **Exercise**—an underused means of increasing and balancing thyroid function. Follow a regular exercise program.

○ **Constitutional hydrotherapy** stimulates the metabolism and thereby stimulates the thyroid gland (see *Appendix A)*.

Impotence

This condition refers to the inability of a male to achieve or maintain an erection. This can be due to physical reasons such as decreased penile blood flow, hormonal imbalance such as low testosterone and the use of certain drugs like hypertension medications, or due to emotional triggers, such as stress.

Nutrition

○ If the impotence has been determined to be due to inadequate blood flow due to arteriosclerosis then following a **plant-based diet**, or one that is quite close to this is highly advisable. One should restrict the intake of red meat as it contains harmful saturated fat.

○ The **intake of fruit and vegetables should be dramatically increased**.

○ **Water soluble fiber** lowers cholesterol which improves blood vessel health—increase intake of oat bran, pectin containing foods such as apples, and rice bran.

○ **Increase fiber**—add high fiber foods to the diet such as apples, oat bran, broccoli, Brussels sprouts, cabbage, carrots, wholegrain flour and green leafy vegetables

○ **Increase water intake**—drink at least six to eight glasses of purified water daily.

○ **Avoid** sugar products, fatty foods and dairy products.

○ Use **cold-pressed oils** such as extra-virgin olive oil or flaxseed oil. If you must fry, *never allow the oil to smoke*—use a medium heat and use extra-virgin olive oil or a heat resistant oil such as cold-pressed peanut or sesame oil. For baking at temperatures above 350°F use butter.

○ Eat **cold water fish** such as mackerel, herring and salmon because they contain essential fatty acids for artery health.

○ Eat **garlic, onions** and **legumes** liberally because they help detoxify the arteries.

○ **Avoid** caffeine, alcohol and tobacco because they interfere with penile blood flow.

○ **Pumpkin seeds**—consume 1/2 cup daily for zinc and essential fatty acids.

Herbal

● **Ginkgo** (24% standardized extract)—improves penile blood flow. Take 80 mg three times daily.

○ **Yohimbe**—used as an aphrodisiac and to increase penile blood flow. Average dosage is 5 mg or 30 drops of extract three times daily. Take under supervision of a physician.

○ **Saw palmetto** (85% to 95% fatty acids and sterols)—used as a tonic for the male reproductive system. Take 160 mg or 30 drops twice daily.

○ **Siberian ginseng** (0.4% eleutherosides)—helps the body adapt to stress. Known to increase libido in some men. Take 250 mg of extract daily or 30 to 60 drops three times daily.

○ **Passion flower**—used as a mild agent to calm the nerves. Take 30 drops four times daily and 60 drops thirty minutes before intercourse.

Vitamins and Minerals

*If **arteriosclerosis** is a problem follow the guidelines in the atheroclerosis section.*

Other

○ **Orchic glandular**—take 1 tablet three times daily between meals to help with testosterone function.

○ **DHEA**—taking 25 to 50 mg daily may increase libido and restore testosterone levels (consult with your physician).

○ **Testosterone**—have your hormone level checked.

○ **Homeopathic Rescue Remedy**—helps with stress related impotency. Take 10 drops before sexual intercourse.

○ **Exercise**—to promote circulation and reduce stress level.

○ Consider **counseling** from a qualified practitioner.

○ Consider **acupuncture** from a qualified practitioner.

○ Consider **homeopathy** from a qualified practitioner.

○ **High blood pressure medication**—impotency is a possible side-effect. Check with your physician.

Indigestion

This is a general term that refers to abdominal cramps, bloating and other discomforts related to inefficient digestion. It is a very common problem in our society of fast foods and high stress. The key to improvement is:

• use natural medicines that stimulate and tonify the digestive organs
• avoid foods that are hard to digest
• reduce stress

Nutrition

● Pay attention to **food sensitivities**—common ones are dairy, wheat, citrus fruit and nuts (see **Elimination and Reintroduction Diet** *Appendix E*).

○ **Minimize fatty foods**, fast foods and deep fried foods.

○ **Avoid** foods with preservatives and artificial sweeteners.

○ **Avoid** caffeine, alcohol, tobacco and refined sugar.

○ **Eat large amounts of vegetables.**

Herbal

● **Peppermint tea**—for treatment and prevention. This herb has a very soothing and anti-inflammatory effect on the digestive system.

O **Chamomile tea**—very soothing, if stress is involved.

To improve digestion use the following herbs for a course of one to two months:

● **Ginger root**—excellent herb to improve digestion and reduce abdominal gas/bloating. Take 1 capsule or 30 drops at beginning of each meal. The tea is also a potent medicine.

O **Gentian root**—stimulates the stomach and other digestive organs to work more efficiently. Take 1 capsule or 30 drops at beginning of each meal.

O **Dandelion root**—helps liver and gall-bladder break down fats. Take 1 capsule or 30 drops at beginning of each meal.

Vitamins and Minerals

O **Multi-vitamin without iron**—take daily for general support.

Other

● **Plant enzymes**—these naturally occurring enzymes help break down food. Take as directed on container with meals.

O **Acidophilus**—take twice daily to fortify the beneficial bacteria that help to metabolize and break down food.

O **Betaine HCl**—take one to two tablets with meals to assist stomach digestion.

O **Homeopathic *Mag phos* 6x**—alleviates stomach cramps associated with indigestion. Take a dose every five minutes until cramps resolve.

O **Homeopathic *Nux vomica* 30C**—helps if stomach pain occurs. Take a dose every half-hour to resolve symptoms.

O **Constitutional hydrotherapy**—see *Appendix A*.

O **Eat in a relaxed atmosphere**.

O **Chew food thoroughly**.

Insomnia

This condition occurs when one wakes frequently throughout the night, wakes up too early or has trouble falling asleep. There are various causes including anxiety, lifestyle habits and slow environmental adaptation.

Nutrition

- **Avoid caffeine**—coffee, black tea, chocolate and soda pops.
- ○ **Avoid alcohol** as it interferes with the quality of sleep.
- ○ **Avoid nicotine** because it is a stimulant.
- ○ **Eat a source of complex carbohydrates before bed.** This helps to stabilize blood sugar levels which may be causing insomnia. Bedtime snacks include wholegrain breads, cereals, muffins and pasta dishes.

Herbal

- **Valerian**—well known for its relaxing effects and not commonly known to cause side-effects. Used for more serious cases of insomnia. Take 2 capsules (150 to 300 mg) or 60 drops half an hour to an hour before bedtime.
- ○ **Passion flower** (4:1 extract)—a more gentle but effective herbal relaxant that helps promote sleep. Take 2 capsules or 60 drops half an hour to an hour before bedtime.
- ○ Other useful herbal medicines for insomnia include **hops** and **skullcap**.

Vitamins and Minerals

- **Calcium** and **magnesium**—this combination has a relaxing effect on the body, especially when taken in the evening. Take 1,000 mg with the evening meal.
- ○ **B complex**—take a 50 mg complex daily. **Vitamin B6** is particularly important for proper sleep.

Other

- Consider **acupuncture** treatments.
- **Foot hydrotherapy**—perform immediately before bedtime for its relaxing effect (see *Appendix A*).
- ○ **Melatonin**—a hormone that regulates the sleep cycle. Start

with 0.3 mg one hour before bedtime and work up to 5 mg if necessary to promote sleep.

○ **Homeopathic *Kali phos* 3x**—take a dose three times daily to help with stress.

○ **Constitutional hydrotherapy**—perform half an hour before bedtime for relaxing effect (see *Appendix A)*.

○ **Daily exercise** leads to improved sleep.

○ **Mental imagery**—imagine a relaxing scene in your mind before trying to fall asleep.

Irritable Bowel Syndrome (IBS)

This syndrome is characterized by abdominal discomfort that can include constipation or diarrhea, or alternate between these two symptoms. As well, mucus formation and bloating are common. Irregular muscle contractions and irritation of the digestive tract lining leads to malabsorption of food and nutrients. The cause is different for each individual but when stress reduction, diet modification and other natural therapies are employed, a cure can occur.

Nutrition

● Pay attention to **food sensitivities**—common ones are dairy, wheat, citrus fruit and nuts. If you feel you are sensitive to one or more of these foods, avoid them for two weeks and see if your digestion improves (see *Appendix E)*.

● **Avoid** foods and substances that irritate the digestive tract such as caffeine, alcohol, tobacco and refined sugars.

○ **Minimize fatty foods**, fast foods and deep fried foods.

○ **Avoid** foods with preservatives and artificial sweeteners.

○ Take a **fiber supplement** that has psyllium seed husks as the base of the formula. Take as directed on container. Drink at least eight ounces of purified water with each dose.

○ **Increase water intake**—drink at least six to eight glasses of purified water daily.

○ Eat a **high fiber diet** that includes lots of vegetables (preferably steamed) and fruit.

Herbal

● **Peppermint tea** or **enteric coated capsules**—used in the treatment and prevention of IBS. This herb has a soothing and anti-inflammatory effect on the digestive system. Take throughout the day.

○ **Chamomile tea**—also used as an anti-inflammatory herb for the digestive tract (especially if stress is involved). Drink throughout the day.

○ **Flaxseed oil**—provides essential fatty acids that promote healthy colon tissue. Take 1 tablespoon daily.

To improve digestion use the following herbs for a course of one to two months:

● **Ginger root**—excellent herb to improve digestion and reduce abdominal gas or bloating. Take 1 capsule or 30 drops at beginning of each meal. Tea can also be used—take 1 cup with meals.

● **Plant enzymes**—these natural enzymes help the body break down food. Take as directed on container with meals.

○ **Dandelion root**—helps liver and gall-bladder to break down fats. Take 1 capsule or 30 drops at beginning of each meal.

○ **Gentian root**—stimulates the stomach and other digestive organs to work more efficiently. Take 1 capsule or 30 drops at beginning of each meal.

Vitamins and Minerals

○ **L-Glutamine**—used for regeneration of the cells of the digestive tract. Take 500 mg twice daily on an empty stomach with water or juice (not milk).

○ **Multi-vitamin without iron**—take daily for general support.

○ **B complex**—stress vitamins. Take a 50 mg complex once daily.

Other

● **Constitutional hydrotherapy**—half an hour before bedtime for relaxation and improved digestion (see *Appendix A*).

● Consider **homeopathy** from a qualified practitioner.

○ **Acidophilus**—take twice daily to strengthen the beneficial bacteria that help to metabolize and break down food.

○ **Fructo-oligosaccharides**—also help to promote beneficial bacteria. Take as directed on container.

○ **Homeopathic *Kali phos* 3x**—take a dose three times daily for stress.

○ **Daily exercise** reduces stress.

○ **Mental imagery**—imagine a relaxing scene while falling asleep.

○ Consider **acupuncture** and **Chinese herbal medicine**.

Jet Lag

This occurs as the body's internal clock (circadian rhythm) adjusts to different time zones. Also, the stress of being in a new place and energy expended while flying leads to difficulty adapting to a new environment.

Nutrition

○ The most important nutritional concern is to **maintain water intake**. When flying the altitude dehydrates you faster than you can notice. Drink one eight-ounce glass of **purified water** every one to two hours.

○ **Avoid dehydrating drinks** such as coffee, soda and alcohol.

Herbal

● **Siberian ginseng** (0.4% eleutherosides)—supports the stress glands in adapting to a new environment. Take 250 mg or 30 drops twice daily. Begin ginseng four days before a long flight, take during the flight and for four days after to keep up energy levels.

○ *Avena sativa*—take 1 capsule or 30 drops three times daily
to help support the nervous system while flying.

Vitamins and Minerals

● **B complex**—helps body to cope with stress at a biochemical
level. Take a 100 mg complex daily.

○ **High potency multi-vitamin**—take daily to protect against
infection and radiation exposure while flying.

○ **Vitamin C with bioflavonoids**—suceptibility to illness
increases while flying. An extra 2,000 to 3,000 mg helps to
support the immune system deal with the increased stress.

Other

● **Homeopathic Rescue Remedy**—take a dose every half-
hour while flying to calm nerves.

● **Melatonin**—used to help normalize the body's biorhythms.
Take 0.5 to 5 mg for the first five evenings at your new
destination.

○ Try to **mimic the anticipated time change** a few days
before arriving in a different time zone.

○ **Homeopathic *Gelsemium* 30C**—take a dose just before
traveling, during travel and upon arrival at destination.

Kidney Stones

These stones are formed by the saturation of urine with either
calcium oxalate (most common), uric acid or phosphates. When
the concentration is too high, these substances can crystallize to
form stones. Natural medicine offers a preventative approach to
this problem and can often help prevent recurrences. Treatment
of chronic or acute kidney stone discomfort must be under the
supervision of a physician.

Nutrition

*To minimize the chances of forming kidney stones one should
consider the following nutritional guidelines:*

● Drink a minimum of six to eight glasses of **purified water daily** to keep urine dilute.

● Consider following a **plant-based diet**, or one low in animal protein, low in fat and high in fiber.

○ **Avoid foods high in oxalate**—beans, cocoa, coffee, parsley, rhubarb, spinach and tea.

○ **Avoid** salt, sugar, alcohol, milk and caffeine.

○ **Increase intake** of foods with a high magnesium to calcium ratio such as barley, bran, corn, buckwheat, soy, rye, oats, brown rice, banana, beans, avocado and potato.

○ Drink **fresh fruit** and **vegetable juices** daily to help normalize urinary pH balance.

Herbal

○ **Cranberry**—cleans out the urinary system. Drink two to four glasses (unsweetened juice) or take a 500 mg cranberry extract tablet (18:1) twice daily.

○ **Rose hip tea**—drink daily as it can be beneficial in reducing kidney stone formation.

Vitamins and Minerals

● **Vitamin B6**—take 50 mg daily with a meal. It helps to break down oxalic acid in the body.

● **Magnesium**—helps with proper metabolism of **calcium**. Take 500 mg twice daily.

○ **B complex**—taken daily along **with extra vitamin B6** to help with proper metabolic processing.

○ **Zinc**—helps to prevent the formation of crystals in the urine. Take a daily total of 50 mg daily with a meal.

○ **Vitamin C with bioflavonoids**—limit intake to 1,000 mg daily.

Other

○ **Homeopathic *Berberis* 30C**—helps alleviate acute pains that radiate from the affected kidney. Take a dose every five minutes for acute relief of kidney stone pain.

○ **Constitutional hydrotherapy**—useful to help detoxify the body as well as improve the efficiency of the urinary system (see *Appendix A*).

○ Consider **acupuncture** and **Chinese herbal medicine** from a qualified practitioner.

○ Have your physician test you for **cadmium—a toxic heavy metal** which can predispose one to kidney stone formation.

Lupus

This is an inflammatory disease where the immune system attacks its own tissues (autoimmune disease). The cause of this reaction is unknown but hormone imbalance, genetics and an undetected viral infection are current theories. The most common form of lupus is known as SLE (Systemic *Lupus erythematosus*). Common symptoms include a butterfly shaped rash over the cheeks and nose, arthritic pains in the joints and scaly red lesions on various parts of the body. Progression of this illness can lead to serious complications in the kidneys, heart, spleen, lungs, brain and other organs.

Nutrition

● Eat a **plant-based diet** with fresh fruit and vegetables daily.

● Identify and eliminate **food allergies** and **sensitivities** (see *Appendix E*).

○ **Avoid** caffeine, dairy, alcohol, sugar and tobacco products.

○ **Reduce or eliminate** the intake of **red meat**.

○ **Fresh fruit** and **vegetable juices** are excellent. Drink daily.

Herbal

○ **Gentian root**—promotes proper absorption of foods. Take 1 capsule or 30 drops with meals.

○ **Licorice root** (12% glycyrrhizin)—supports the stress glands and is a natural anti-inflammatory. Take 1,000 to 1,500 mg of **deglycyrrhizinated** licorice root or 30 drops of extract three times daily.

○ **Milk thistle** (80% standardized extract)—detoxifies the liver and blood. Take 300 mg daily.

○ **Flaxseed oil**—supplies essential fatty acids that decrease inflammation. Take 1 tablespoon twice daily.

○ **Plant enzymes**—take daily with meals to promote proper digestion and metabolism. Take as directed on container.

Vitamins and Minerals

○ **High potency multi-vitamin without iron**—take daily to ensure against nutritional deficiencies.

○ **Vitamin B12**—protective effect on nervous system. Take 2 mg daily or have 1 mg injected twice weekly by a physician.

○ **Vitamin C with bioflavonoids**—supports the stress glands and immune system. Take 1,000 mg three times daily.

○ **Grape seed extract (PCO)**—a potent antioxidant to support the immune system. Take 50 mg twice daily.

○ **Vitamin E**—a natural anti-inflammatory. Take 800 IU daily.

Other

● **DHEA**—this hormone has shown promise in short-term studies in reducing inflammation associated with lupus. Have levels measured by a physician. Dosage can range from 10 to 1,000 mg daily.

● Consider **homeopathy** from a qualified practitioner.

● Consider **acupuncture** and **Chinese herbal medicine** from a qualified practitioner.

● **Hormone balance** is very important. Consult with a physician trained in natural medicine about your hormone status.

○ **Pregnenolone**—a precursor to hormones. Talk to your physician about its use. Typical dosage is 10 to 200 mg daily

○ **Constitutional hydrotherapy**—see *Appendix A*.

Menopause

This refers to a transitional time (averaging at age 50) in a woman's life when the ovaries begin to reduce production of estrogen and progesterone. As a result, some women experience symptoms such as hot flashes, irregular uterine bleeding, fatigue, vaginal dryness and mood changes. Bone loss can accelerate at this time as hormone levels decrease. I have found natural medicine works extremely well to help the body adjust to this transition and to relieve symptoms. A small percentage of women require hormone replacement therapy.

Nutrition

● Focus on **a plant-based diet**. Consume unprocessed foods, fruits, vegetables, whole grains, and **foods high in calcium** (see *Osteoporosis* section for a list of high-calcium foods).

● **Soy products** are excellent to consume as they contain genistein, which appears to have hormone balancing qualities.

○ **Avoid** high salt intake, alcohol, smoking and sugar products.

○ **Eat** foods low in fat and high in fiber.

○ **Decrease** intake of red meat, dairy products and caffeine.

Herbal

The following herbs can be effective in alleviating menopausal symptoms. Look for formulas that contain a similar blend of herbs or take them individually.

● **Angelica/Dong quai**—take 2 capsules or 30 drops twice daily.

● **Black cohosh**—take 2 capsules or 30 drops twice daily.

○ **Licorice root**—take 2 capsules or 30 drops twice daily.

○ **Wild yam** *(Dioscorea)*—take 2 capsules or 30 drops twice daily.

○ **Vitex**—take 2 capsules or 30 drops twice daily.

○ **Evening primrose oil**—contains essential fatty acids which help to relieve menopausal symptoms. Take as directed on container.

○ **Flaxseed oil**—contains essential fatty acids used as hormonal precursors. Take 1 to 2 tablespoons daily.

Vitamins and Minerals

● **Vitamin E**—alleviates hot flashes and vaginal dryness. Take 800 to 1200 IU daily with meals.

○ **High potency multi-vitamin without iron**—take daily. If anemia is a problem take a multi-vitamin with iron.

○ **Calcium**—to prevent bone loss 1,000 mg should be taken daily with a meal.

○ **Magnesium**—to prevent bone loss take 500 to 1,000 mg daily.

Other

● Consider **homeopathy** from a qualified practitioner.

○ Consider the use of **DHEA** supplementation with the supervision of your physician at a dosage of 20 to 50 mg daily.

○ **Testosterone** may be needed for low libido. Consult with your physician about its use.

○ **Glandular treatment**—to tonify the hormonal glands and help balance hormone levels. These include thyroid, adrenal, pituitary, ovary and uterus glandulars, or glandular formulas.

○ Consider **acupuncture** and **Chinese herbal medicine** from a qualified practitioner.

○ Consider the use of **natural progesterone**. Talk to your physician.

Menstrual Cramps

Cramping pain occurs when the uterus contracts forcefully or when clots are passed through the uterus during menstrual flow. Pain may be felt throughout the abdomen and lower back. Natural medicine works well for acute menstrual cramps and to remove the long-term susceptibility to them. Hormonal imbalance is the underlying cause of this condition.

Nutrition

○ **Avoid caffeine** products because they can worsen existing cramps. These products include chocolate, black tea, soda pop and coffee.

Herbal

- **Crampbark**—an antispasmodic and pain reliever for the uterus. Take 2 capsules or 30 drops of extract every thirty minutes until symptoms subside.
- **Blue cohosh**—an antispasmodic and pain reliever for the uterus. Take 2 capsules or 30 drops of extract every thirty minutes until symptoms subside
- ○ **Raspberry leaf**—relaxes the uterus. Take 2 capsules, 60 drops or 1 cup of tea every half-hour until symptoms subside.
- ○ **Flaxseed oil**—decreases inflammation by supplying essential fatty acids. Take 1 tablespoon daily.
- ○ **Valerian root**—an antispasmodic for the uterus and relaxes the nervous system. Take two 300 mg capsules or 60 drops every two hours until symptoms subside.

For prevention of menstrual cramps:
- **Wild yam cream**—a source of natural progesterone. Apply as directed on container for the last fourteen days of the menstrual cycle and discontinue when menstrual flow starts.
- ○ **Angelica/Dong quai** (4:1 extract)—to balance the menstrual cycle take 2 capsules (125 mg each) or 30 drops of extract twice daily until menses start.
- ○ **Dandelion root**—for liver tonification (the liver helps the body to metabolize hormones properly) take 2 capsules twice daily.
- ○ **Evening primrose oil**—supplies essential fatty acids that have natural anti-inflammatory properties. Take daily as directed on container.

Vitamins and Minerals

- ○ **Calcium**—a muscle relaxant for the uterus. Take 1,000 mg daily with a meal.
- ○ **Magnesium**—a muscle relaxant for the uterus. Take 500 to 1,000 mg daily with a meal.
- ○ **B complex**—useful in preventing cramps. Take a 50 mg complex daily.
- ○ **Vitamin E**—a natural anti-inflammatory. Take 800 IU daily with a meal.

Other

- **Homeopathic *Mag phos* 6x**—take a dose every fifteen minutes until symptoms subside (see *Appendix B*).
- **Constitutional hydrotherapy**—works quickly to relieve congestion of blood in the pelvic area which helps to decrease pain (see *Appendix A*).
- ○ Consider **acupuncture** from a practitioner. It works well for acute menstrual cramps and for long-term prevention.
- ○ Consider **homeopathy** from a practitioner. It works well for acute menstrual cramps and for long-term prevention.

Multiple Sclerosis

This is a degenerative disorder where the immune system attacks and damages areas of the nervous system. Symptoms vary depending on which areas are affected and can include muscle weakness, abnormal sensations throughout the body, vision loss, light-headedness, urinary incontinence and digestive upset. The exact cause is unknown and there may be a complex of causative factors. I have seen comprehensive naturopathic protocols to be beneficial for this condition.

Nutrition

- Identify and eliminate **food allergies** and **sensitivities** (see *Appendix E*).
- ○ The **Swank Diet** developed by neurologist Roy Swank, MD, is a long-standing traditional dietary treatment for MS— follow these guidelines:
  - saturated fat intake of less than 10 g per day
  - daily intake of 40 to 50 g of polyunsaturated oils
  - no margarine or hydrogenated oils
  - 1 teaspoon of cod liver oil daily
  - consume fish four or more times weekly

- ○ Eat **cold water fish** which are excellent sources of omega-3 oils which help in normal nerve function. These include mackerel, herring and salmon.

○ **Avoid** dairy products, refined sugars, caffeine, tobacco and alcohol.

○ Use **cold-pressed oils** such as extra-virgin olive oil or flaxseed oil. If you must fry, *never allow the oil to smoke*—use a medium heat and use extra-virgin olive oil or a heat resistant oil such as cold-pressed peanut or sesame oil. For baking at temperatures above 350°F use butter.

○ Include **extra-virgin olive oil** in the diet.

Herbal

● **Flaxseed oil**—supplies essential fatty acids for nerve health. Take 1 tablespoon daily or 1 capsule three times daily.

● **Black currant oil**—supplies essential fatty acids for nerve health. Take 1 capsule three times daily.

○ **Licorice root** (12% glycyrrhizin)—a natural anti-inflammatory. Take 1 capsule or 30 drops three times daily.

○ **Curcuma**—a natural anti-inflammatory. Take 200 mg of standardized curcuma twice daily.

○ **Ginkgo**—enhances circulation to the muscles and nerves of the body. Take 60 mg three times daily.

Vitamins and Minerals

● **Vitamin B12 and folic acid**—very specific for regeneration of nerve tissue. Have your physician give you an injection of these B vitamins on a weekly basis.

○ **B complex**—for nerve health. Take a 100 mg B complex daily.

○ **High potency multi-vitamin without iron**—take daily to ensure against nutritional deficiencies.

○ **Selenium**—an antioxidant that protects nerve tissue. Take 200 mcg daily.

○ **Grape seed extract (PCO)**—an antioxidant that protects nerve tissue. Take 50 mg three times daily.

○ **Vitamin E**—an antioxidant that protects nerve tissue. Take 800 IU daily.

○ **Calcium and magnesium**—needed for proper nerve function. Take 1,000 mg of each with a meal.

Other

- **Stress reduction** techniques—exercise, yoga, t'ai chi and mental imagery.
- Consider **homeopathy** from a qualified practitioner.
- Consider **acupuncture** from a qualified practitioner.
- ○ **Exercise** on a regular basis.
- ○ **Homeopathic *Kali phos* 6x**—supports the nervous system. Take a dose three times daily.
- ○ **Homeopathic *Mag phos* 6x**—supports the nervous system. Take a dose three times daily.
- ○ **Adrenal glandular**—supports the stress glands. Take 1 tablet three times daily.
- ○ **DHEA**—is proving to be useful for its anti-inflammatory effects. Have your levels tested and supplemented if needed by your physician. An average adult dosage is 20 to 100 mg daily.
- ○ **Pregnenolone**—is proving to be useful for its anti-inflammatory effects. Have your levels tested and supplemented as needed by your physician.
- ○ **Salmon oil**—supplies omega-3 fatty acids for nerve and artery health. Take 2 capsules (1,000 mg each) twice daily.

Muscle Cramps

These are painful contractions of the muscle fibers. The calves of the legs are most commonly affected. Muscle cramps in children are generally related to a calcium and magnesium imbalance. Cramps in adults are generally due to poor circulation or nutritional deficiencies like zinc, vitamin E, calcium and magnesium. Dehydration and imbalanced levels of sodium and potassium can also lead to muscle cramps.

Nutrition

- ○ **Eat** a diet low in refined sugars and alcohol.
- ○ **Avoid** tobacco and caffeine as they interfere with circulation.
- ○ Eat **smaller, more frequent meals** as low blood sugar may trigger muscle cramps.

○ Eat **calcium-rich foods** such as yogurt, broccoli, sesame seeds, tofu, sardines and collard greens.

○ Eat **magnesium-rich foods** such as fish, nuts, green vegetables, whole wheat, bananas, grapes, peaches, plums, pumpkin, potatoes, beets and zucchini.

Herbal

● **Ginkgo** (24% standardized extract)—excellent for improving circulation in the limbs. Take an 80 mg capsule or 30 drops of extract twice daily.

○ **Stinging nettle**—has a high mineral content that is useful for this condition. Take 1 capsule or 30 drops three times daily.

○ **Ginger**—promotes circulation throughout the tissues. Take a 250 mg capsule twice daily or drink ginger tea throughout the day.

○ **Cinnamon tea**—dilates blood vessels and promotes circulation. Drink throughout the day.

○ **Cayenne**—well known for its ability to enhance circulation. Take as directed on container.

Vitamins and Minerals

The following vitamins are useful and all may be found in one formula:

● **Calcium**—take 1,000 mg with evening meal.

● **Magnesium**—take 1,000 mg with evening meal.

● **High potency multi-vitamin without iron**—take daily to ensure against nutritional deficiencies.

○ **Vitamin E**—take 400 to 800 IU daily.

○ **Zinc**—take 50 mg daily **with** 3 mg of **copper**.

○ **B complex**—take a 50 mg complex once daily.

Other

● **Homeopathic *Mag phos* 6x** and ***Calc phos* 6x**—for efficient utilization of calcium and magnesium. Take a dose of each three times daily away from meals.

- **Foot hydrotherapy**—see *Appendix A.*
- ○ Consider **acupuncture** from a qualified practitioner.

Nausea

This condition can be caused by motion sickness, pregnancy, food poisoning, food sensitivity, or mental and emotional factors. Persistent nausea should be medically evaluated.

Nutrition

- **Suspect foods should be eliminated** from the diet for two weeks and slowly re-introduced to see if they cause symptoms to recur. See **Elimination and Reintroduction Diet** *(Appendix E)*.
- ○ **Decrease dairy intake** as it is a common food sensitivity with this condition.

Herbal

- **Ginger**—well known and researched for its ability to fight nausea. Take a 250 mg capsule or 30 drops three times daily. Ginger tea is also excellent.
- ○ **Dandelion root**—improves liver and digestive function which can help alleviate nausea. Take 1 capsule or 30 drops with meals.

Vitamins and Minerals

- ○ **Vitamin B6**—take 50 mg daily (can be in the form of a **B complex**).

Other

- **Homeopathic *Ipecac* 30C**—take a dose every one to two hours for acute nausea.
- **Homeopathic *Nux vomica* 30C**—used when nausea is the result of bad food or from hangover. Take a dose every one to two hours for acute relief of symptoms.

○ Consider **acupuncture** from a qualified practitioner.

○ Regular **exercise**—partake in aerobic exercise three times weekly.

Osteoporosis

This condition is characterized by a decrease in normal bone density. There are multiple factors involved in the development of osteoporosis such as nutritional status, digestive function, hormonal status, environment and lifestyle habits. Postmenopausal women are at greatest risk for complications from osteoporosis, although the cycle of events leading up to the loss in bone density begins many years before it is diagnosed. This illness leads to a higher likelihood of fractures due to the porous bone structure.

Nutritional

● **Avoid** foods and products that increase the excretion of calcium: caffeine, sugar products, alcohol, smoking, soda pop and salt.

● The following foods are good **sources of calcium**:

Food Amount	Calcium Content
sardines 3 ounces	375 mg
yogurt 1 cup (eight ounces)	357 mg
collard greens 1 cup packed	355 mg
whole milk 1 cup	288 mg
sesame seeds 1/4 cup	250 mg
turnip greens 1 cup	250 mg
broccoli 1 cup	180 mg
almonds 2 ounces	150 mg
beans 1 cup	150 mg
blackstrap molasses 1 tablespoon	150 mg
kale 1 cup	150 mg
salmon (canned) 3 ounces	150 mg
tofu 4 ounces	150 mg
apricots (dried) 1 cup	100 mg

○ **Avoid** a diet high in animal protein.

○ Eat **whole grains** such as brown rice, oats, millet, barley, spelt, amaranth and quinoa.

○ Consume **soy foods**—they contain the chemicals dadzein and genistein that stop bone demineralization.

Herbal

Digestive herbs are used to increase the stomach acid so that calcium can be absorbed properly from food and vitamin supplements. Efficient digestion is a must for proper absorption.

● **Gentian root**—take 1 capsule or 30 drops at each meal.

○ **Dandelion root**—take 1 capsule or 30 drops at beginning of each meal.

Vitamins and Minerals

● Many **vitamins and minerals** are known to be important in the prevention and reversal of bone loss. These include:

Supplement	Daily Amount
boron	.3 mg
copper	.3 mg
folic acid	400–1,000 mcg
manganese	10–20 mg
silicon	1 mg
strontium	.5–3 mg
vitamin B6	.50 mg
vitamin C	1,000 mg twice daily
vitamin D	400 IU
vitamin K	200–400 mcg
zinc	30 mg

*Note: **Vitamin K** is measured in mg, not g. Check with your physician before starting this program to make sure it does not interfere with any medications you are using. For example, vitamin K interferes with blood thinning drugs.*

Also: **Magnesium** *in excessive amounts may cause diarrhea. If this occurs, cut back on the dosage and then gradually increase the amount to a comfortable level.*

● **Calcium**—an integral component for bone formation. Take 500 mg twice daily with meals.

● **Magnesium**—an essential component for bone formation. Take 500 mg twice daily with meals.

● **High potency multi-vitamin without iron**—take daily to ensure against nutritional deficiencies.

Other

● **Betaine HCl**—take 1 to 2 tablets at each meal to aid digestion.

● **Avoid smoking** as it accelerates bone loss.

● Engage in **weight-bearing exercise** such as walking, running and weight lifting for half an hour three to five times weekly.

● **Homeopathic *Calc phos* 6x**—take a dose three times daily.

○ **DHEA**—beneficial to reverse bone loss. Consult with your physician about its use. Average dosage is 10 to 50 mg daily.

○ **Homeopathic *Calc fluor* 6x**—take a dose three times daily.

○ **Natural progesterone cream**—talk to your holistic doctor about the use of natural progesterone cream. Recent studies have shown it to be effective in the treatment of osteoporosis. Use alone or in conjunction with estrogen if needed.

Pink Eye (Conjunctivitis)

This conditions refers to an inflammation of the conjunctiva (membrane that lines the inside of the eyelid and outside lining of the eyeball). The eyes often become bloodshot and swollen due to the irritation. Common causes include bacterial or viral infections, or environmental causes such as allergies, wind and chemicals or other foreign substances. Infection caused by a virus can be quite contagious. A medical professional should be seen to rule out serious eye conditions.

Nutrition

○ **Avoid** alcohol, tobacco, sugar and caffeine products.

○ Eat **beets** and **carrots** or drink their juice for nutrients beneficial for eye health.

Herbal

● **Eyewash**—in an ounce container, add 20 drops each of goldenseal tincture and eyebright tincture. Fill the rest of the container with non-injectable saline solution. Shake to mix the solution. Put 2 drops into the affected eye every two hours for severe infections.

○ **Eyebright** (4:1 extract)—can be taken internally or used topically. Take 2 capsules or 60 drops four times daily until condition resolves.

○ **Echinacea** (4% echinacosides and 0.7% flavonoids)—take 2 capsules or 60 drops three times daily.

○ **Stinging nettle**—if there is an allergic component take 2 capsules or 60 drops four times daily.

Vitamins and Minerals

● **Vitamin A**—promotes healing. Take 25,000 IU daily until condition resolves (*avoid if pregnant*).

● **Vitamin C with bioflavonoids**—stimulates the immune system and is anti-allergenic. Take 3,000 to 5,000 mg daily.

○ **Beta-carotene**—promotes healing. Take 100,000 IU daily.

○ **Quercitin**—for allergic reaction take 500 mg three times daily.

Other

● Apply **alternating hot** (30 secs) **and cold** (30 secs) **compresses** to the eye. Repeat three times and perform every two hours.

○ **Homeopathic** *Euphrasia* **30C**—specific for conjunctivitis when the eyes are red and itchy. Take a dose every two hours until symptoms subside.

○ **Homeopathic** *Pulsatilla* **30C**—specific for conjunctivitis when the eyes have yellowish-green, sticky discharge. Take a dose every two hours until symptoms subside.

○ **Avoid touching** and contaminating non-infected eye as conjunctivitis is **very contagious**.

○ **Foot hydrotherapy**—see *Appendix A.*

PMS (Premenstrual Syndrome)

Premenstrual syndrome is a complex of symptoms experienced seven to fourteen days prior to menstruation. These symptoms may include mood swings, decreased energy, water retention, altered sex drive, breast pain, backache and headache.

Nutrition

○ **Reduce intake** of refined sugar, salt, fatty foods, caffeine, alcohol and tobacco.

○ Eat **organic meat** as it does not contain artificial hormones.

○ **Eat** a diet high in **fish, vegetables** and **fruit.**

○ Take a **fiber supplement** composed of psyllium seed husks daily as it helps bind excess estrogen, a major female hormone that may cause PMS symptoms. Drink a large glass of purified water with each dose.

○ Identify and eliminate **food allergies** and **sensitivities** (see *Appendix E*).

Herbal

The following herbs are used for hormone balancing:

● **Vitex**—take 1 capsule or 30 drops twice daily until menses start, then discontinue.

○ **Licorice root** (12% glycyrrhizin)—take 1 capsule or 30 drops three times daily.

○ **Crampbark**—take 1 capsule or 30 drops twice daily.

○ **Angelica/Dong quai** (4:1 extract)—take 2 capsules (125 mg each) twice daily until menses start, then discontinue.

The liver is involved in metabolizing hormones and needs to be working optimally to improve PMS. *The following herbs are used to improve liver function:*

- **Dandelion root**—take 1 capsule or 30 drops three times daily.
- ○ **Milk thistle** (80% silymarin)—take a daily total of 250 mg or 30 drops with each meal.

Vitamins and Minerals

- **Magnesium**—often deficient in this condition. Take 500 mg with evening meal.
- **B complex**—helps body deal with stress and metabolize hormones. Take a 50 mg complex once daily.
- ○ **Calcium**—take 1,000 mg with evening meal.
- ○ **Vitamin E**—useful if breast tenderness is a problem. Take 400 to 800 IU daily.
- ○ **Evening primrose oil**—supplies essential fatty acids for proper hormone balance. Take 1 capsule three times daily.
- ○ **Vitamin B6**—known to help alleviate PMS. Take a daily total of 100 to 150 mg.

Other

- ○ **Daily exercise** is useful. Follow a consistent exercise program.
- ○ **Natural progesterone cream**—taken from ovulation until the first day of menstrual flow works well in alleviating PMS.
- ○ Consider **homeopathy** from a qualified practitioner.
- ○ Consider **acupuncture** from a qualified practitioner.

Prostate Enlargement

The prostate is a walnut shaped gland located below the bladder in males. If the prostate gland enlarges (hyperplasia) it interferes with the flow of urine. Resulting symptoms may include frequent urination (both day and night), decreased force of urinary stream and difficulty starting and stopping the flow of urine. It appears that as men age the hormones dihydrotestosterone and estrogen stimulate growth of the prostate gland. This condition generally responds extremely well to natural therapy.

Nutrition

○ Eat **pumpkin seeds**—they contain zinc and essential fatty acids for prostate health. Recommended portion: 1/2 cup daily.

○ **Avoid** the following foods that increase inflammation: caffeine (coffee, tea, chocolate and soda pop), alcohol, tobacco and sugar products.

○ **Increase water intake**—drink six to eight glasses of purified water daily.

Herbal

The following herbs shrink and heal the prostate gland. The combination of saw palmetto and pygeum is very effective.

● **Saw palmetto extract** (85% to 95% fatty acids and sterols)—take 160 mg or 30 drops twice daily for at least two months.

○ *Pygeum africanum* (13% total sterols)—take 40 mg twice daily for at least two months.

○ **Flaxseed oil**—supplies essential fatty acids that decrease inflammation. Take 1 tablespoon twice daily.

Vitamins and Minerals

● **Zinc**—essential for prostate health. Take 50 mg daily.

● **Copper**—a balancer for **zinc**. Take 3 mg daily.

○ **Vitamin E**—a natural anti-inflammatory. Take 400 IU daily with a meal.

These amino acids promote health of the prostate gland:

○ **Glycine**—take 200 mg daily between meals.

○ **Glutamic acid**—take 200 mg daily between meals.

○ **Alanine**—take 200 mg daily between meals.

Other

● Consider **acupuncture** and **Chinese herbal medicine** from a qualified practitioner.

O **Homeopathic** *Sabal serrulata* **3x**—specific for men with an enlarged prostate and who are also prone to bladder infections. Take a dose twice daily for at least two months.

O **Exercise**—promotes circulation and reduces swelling.

O Consider **homeopathy** from a qualified practitioner.

O **Constitutional hydrotherapy**—see *Appendix A.*

O **Salmon oil**—supplies fatty acids reducing pain and inflammation in the body. Take 2 capsules (1,000 mg each) twice daily.

Psoriasis

This condition results when the skin cells multiply too quickly leading to an accumulation of skin lesions that have a characteristic reddish base covered with silvery scales. The naturopathic approach is to detoxify the body so that the skin (the body's largest organ of elimination) will not have to eliminate toxins. My experience has been that diet, digestive function and liver function must be addressed in order to resolve this problem.

Nutrition

● Identify and eliminate **food allergies** and **sensitivities** (see *Appendix E*).

O **Minimize** the consumption of the following foods as they can aggravate this condition: red meat, dairy products, fatty foods, sugar, citrus fruits, caffeine and alcohol.

O Consume **fresh fruit** and **vegetable juices** daily.

O Eat **cold water fish** such as mackerel, herring and salmon regularly as they contain essential fatty acids for healthy skin.

O Drink six to eight glasses of **purified water** daily.

O Take a **fiber supplement** composed of psyllium seed husks to promote elimination in the bowels daily. Drink eight ounces of purified water with each dose.

Herbal

● **Burdock root**—helps skin conditions by detoxifying the body. Take 1 capsule or 30 drops three times daily.

- **Plant enzymes**—aid in proper food digestion. Take with meals as directed on container.
- **Sarsaparilla**—a specific herb used in the treatment of psoriasis. Take 1 capsule or 30 drops three times daily for a minimum of two months.
- **Flaxseed oil**—contains essential fatty acids that decrease inflammation. Take 1 to 2 tablespoons daily.
- **Milk thistle** (80% silymarin)—detoxifies the liver. Take 250 mg or 30 drops with each meal..

Vitamins and Minerals

The following vitamins can often be found in a formula:
- **B complex**—take a 50 mg complex twice daily.
- **Zinc**—take 30 mg daily **with** 3 to 4 mg of **copper**.
- **Selenium**—take 200 mcg daily.
- **Vitamin D3 cream**—discuss its use with your dermatologist.
- **High potency multi-vitamin without iron**—take daily to ensure against nutritional deficiencies.

Other

- **Betaine HCl**—improves digestion. Take 1 to 2 tablets with meals.
- **Shark cartilage**—may be beneficial. Take as directed on container.
- **Sunlight** is helpful for some patients.
- **Constitutional hydrotherapy**—see *Appendix A*.
- Consider **homeopathy** from a qualified practitioner.
- Consider **acupuncture** and **Chinese herbal medicine** from a qualified practitioner.
- **Salmon oil**—supplies omega-3 fatty acids for skin health. Take 2 capsules (1,000 mg each) twice daily.

Rash

The skin is the body's largest organ. It functions as a protective barrier against the environment, allows the body to cool off through perspiration and provides a route for elimination of toxins. A rash occurs when there is external irritation (such as a reaction to a deodorant or an irritant like poison ivy), or when internal toxins build up and must be eliminated through the skin. These toxins are generally produced from poor digestive function and consumption of food allergens.

Nutrition

- **Elimination and Reintroduction Diet**—see *Appendix E.*

Herbal

- **Burdock root**—detoxifies the skin. Take 1 capsule or 30 drops three times daily.
- **Flaxseed oil**—provides essential fatty acids for skin health. Take 1 tablespoon daily for a minimum of three months.
- **Gentian root**—improves digestion. Take 1 capsule or 30 drops before each meal.
- **Calendula tincture**—use externally to soothe and heal rashes.
- **Chamomile**—make a tea and then use in a compress over the affected area.

Vitamins and Minerals

- **Vitamin C with bioflavonoids**—a natural anti-inflammatory and detoxifier. Take 3,000 mg daily in divided doses.
- **Beta-carotene**—is anti-allergenic and helps with skin repair. Take 50,000 IU daily.
- **Selenium**—detoxifies the skin. Take a daily total of 200 mcg.
- **Vitamin E**—can be used topically or taken internally at 400 IU daily when dry skin is present.
- **L-Glutathione**—an antioxidant used by the body for detoxification. Take 500 mg twice daily.

Other

- **Constitutional hydrotherapy**—see *Appendix A*.
- ○ **Acidophilus**—supplementation of this friendly bacteria is especially useful if antibiotics have been used.
- ○ **Oatmeal bath**—decreases itching and heals skin—used to relieve acute symptoms. Put half a cup of oatmeal powder into bath and soak for ten to fifteen minutes. Do not rinse after the bath, just pat dry. Repeat daily.
- ○ **Salmon oil**—supplies omega-3 fatty acids for skin health. Take 2 capsules (1,000 mg each) twice daily.

Sinusitis

Sinusitis is an infection or congestion of one or more of the sinuses in the skull. Acute sinusitis can be caused by a viral or bacterial infection and is frequently a complication of an upper respiratory infection such as a cold. Symptoms usually include fever, facial pain and inability to clear the nasal passages. Chronic sinus congestion is generally related to food allergies and sensitivities and tends to have less severe symptoms than acute sinusitis.

Nutrition

- **Food allergies** and **sensitivities** need to be identified and eliminated for resolution of chronic sinusitis (see *Appendix E*).
- ○ **Avoid dairy products** and **bananas** as they produce mucus which can lead to clogging of the sinus.

Herbal

- **Goldenseal**—this herb has a specific action to fight sinus infections. Take 2 capsules or 30 drops four times daily.
- ○ **Horseradish**—stimulates sinus drainage. Eat horseradish or take 10 drops of extract three times daily.
- ○ **Echinacea** (4% echinacosides and 0.7% flavonoids)— stimulates the immune system to fight infections. Take 2 capsules (250 mg each) or 30 drops four times daily.

○ **Ephedra**—herbal formulas that contain ephedra can be used over a short term for relief of acute sinus congestion (*for adults only*).

Vitamins and Minerals

● **Vitamin C with bioflavonoids**—stimulates the immune system. Take 1,000 mg three to four times daily.
● **N-Acetylcysteine**—liquifies mucus so the sinus cavities can drain. Take 500 mg twice daily.
○ **Zinc**—stimulates the immune system. Take 30 mg daily.
○ **Copper**—works in conjunction with **zinc**. Take 3 mg daily.
○ **Grape seed extract (PCO)**—has a powerful effect against allergies. Take 50 mg twice daily.
○ **High potency multi-vitamin without iron**—take daily to optimize immune system function.

Other

● **Facial compress**—to relieve congestion alternate one minute of a warm wet face cloth and thirty seconds of a cold wet face cloth, three times to face.
● **Homeopathic combination sinus formula**.
○ **Steam inhalation**—boil water and then add a few drops of eucalyptus oil. Place towel over the head and lean near the water and breathe deeply. Repeat a couple times daily to relieve sinus congestion.
○ **Homeopathic *Pulsatilla* 30C**—when yellowish-green mucus is present and the sinus feels better in the fresh air this medicine can be very effective. Take a dose twice daily.
○ Consider **homeopathy** from a qualified practitioner.
○ Consider **acupuncture** and **Chinese herbal medicine**.
○ **Foot hydrotherapy**—see *Appendix A*.

Sore Throat

Sore throats are generally caused by viral or bacterial infections, or they may be the result of allergies. Mild to moderate cases can be treated very effectively with natural treatments. Medical consultation is necessary for more severe cases such as the bacterial infection known as strep throat.

Nutrition

○ Eat foods that are easy to digest and do not irritate the throat. These include **soups** and **fresh fruit** and **vegetable juices**.

○ **Avoid foods that lower immune function** such as dairy products and refined sugar products.

Herbal

● **Goldenseal**—has antiviral, antibacterial and immune stimulating properties. Take 60 drops in a glass of warm water, gargle and swallow. One can also take 2 capsules every two hours until symptoms subside.

● **Slippery elm**—very soothing to an inflamed throat. Suck on a slippery elm lozenge as needed for relief of symptoms.

○ **Echinacea** (4% echinacosides and 0.7% flavonoids)—has antiviral, antibacterial and immune stimulating properties. Take 2 capsules (250 mg each) or 30 drops every two hours until symptoms subside.

○ **Garlic**—has antiviral, antibacterial and immune stimulating properties. Take 2 capsules every three hours.

○ **Ginger**—relieves pain in and inflammation of the throat. Take 2 capsules, 30 drops or 1 cup of ginger tea every two hours until symptoms subside.

○ **Marshmallow root**—very soothing to an irritated throat. Take 2 capsules or 30 drops four times daily.

Vitamins and Minerals

● **Vitamin C with bioflavonoids**—stimulates the immune system. Take 1,000 mg three to four times daily.

○ **Beta-carotene**—protects the lining of the respiratory tract. Take 100,000 IU daily.

○ **Zinc lozenges**—can help clear up throat infection. Take lozenge every two hours for acute infection.

○ **Vitamin A**—promotes healing of the throat and respiratory tract. Take 50,000 IU for one week to eliminate a sore throat.

Other

● **Throat compress**—soak a face cloth in cold water, wring it out and lay it over the throat. Place a dry towel over the entire neck area and leave in place for an hour. This acts as a decongestant and stimulates immune cells as the body warms up the cold towel.

○ **Constitutional hydrotherapy**—can be used in conjunction with the throat compress for a more intense treatment (see *Appendix A*).

○ **Foot hydrotherapy**—see *Appendix A*.

○ **Gargling with salt water** (1/2 teaspoon of salt in a glass of warm water) disinfects the throat. Repeat every three hours.

○ **Homeopathic combination sore throat formula**—take as directed on container.

Sprains and Strains

These occur as muscles, tendons, ligaments and other connective tissue become damaged from various causes such as excessive activity or stretching. As a result, pain, swelling, loss of mobility or strength, and spasm may occur.

Nutrition

○ **Avoid** caffeine, alcohol, refined sugar and tobacco products because they hinder the healing process.

Herbal

● **Bromelain**—a natural anti-inflammatory that speeds healing of damaged tissue. Take 500 mg three times daily between meals.

○ **Arnica oil**—decreases pain and inflammation. **Apply externally** to injured areas with unbroken skin (*do not take internally*).

○ **Curcumin**—acts as a natural anti-inflammatory and reduces swelling. Take 2 capsules three times daily.

Vitamins and Minerals

● **Glucosamine sulfate**—used to build connective tissue. Take 500 mg three times daily.
● **Vitamin C with bioflavonoids**—used to build connective tissue. Take 1,000 mg three times daily.
○ **Vitamin E**—is a natural anti-inflammatory and aids in muscle recuperation. Take 400 to 800 IU daily with a meal.
○ **Zinc**—specific nutrient for the formation of connective tissue. Take 30 mg daily **with** 3 mg of **copper**.
○ **Manganese**—specific nutrient for connective tissue repair. Take daily as part of a **high potency multi-vitamin without iron**.

Other

● **RICE**, for the **first twenty-four hours**
  R—Rest the injury.
  I—Ice the injured area for the first 24 to 48 hours.
  C—Compress the area with a bandage for support.
  E—Elevate the injured area for proper circulation.
○ **After twenty-four hours** apply alternating hot and cold compresses to the affected area to speed healing and promote tissue repair.
● Consider **physiotherapy** from a qualified practitioner.
● Consider **acupuncture** from a qualified practitioner.
● **Homeopathic** *Calc fluor* **6x**—builds connective tissue. Take a dose three times daily.
● **Homeopathic** *Arnica* **30C**—take as soon as possible after an injury to minimize swelling and bruising. Take a dose twice daily for three days.
○ **Homeopathic** *Rhus tox* **30C**—specific for connective tissue injuries due to overexertion. Take a dose twice daily until pain, swelling and stiffness is gone.
○ **Homeopathic** *Calc fluor* **6x**—repairs connective tissue, especially for chronic injuries. Take a dose three times daily.

○ **Glandular connective tissue complex**—provides specific nutrients for damaged tissue. Take as directed on container.

○ **Homeopathic *Silicea* 6x**—builds connective tissue. Take a dose three times daily.

Stress

Everyone reacts to mental, physical and emotional stimuli. Stress can be positive or negative depending on how it is perceived. Poor stress coping mechanisms lead to physiological changes that result in illness. Natural therapies enable the mind and body to adapt to and cope with stressors. Try to incorporate natural therapies such as aromatherapy, hydrotherapy, massage, acupuncture and saunas into your lifestyle.

Nutrition

○ **Avoid** refined sugars products, artificial sweeteners, caffeine, alcohol and tobacco. These substances increase the cortisol released by the stress glands thereby depleting these glands and leading to inefficient response to stress.

○ **Increase intake** of fruits, vegetables and whole grains.

○ **Oatmeal** is an excellent tonic for the nervous system.

○ **Fruit** and **vegetable juices** nourish immune and nervous systems.

Herbal

● **Siberian ginseng** (0.4% eleutherosides)—stimulates and nourishes the stress glands. Take 250 mg of standardized extract or 30 drops two to three times daily.

○ **Oatstraw**—an excellent tonic for the nervous system. Take 1 capsule or 30 drops three times daily.

○ **Valerian**—a strong herbal nerve relaxant. Take 300 mg or 30 drops two to three times daily.

○ **Chamomile tea**—an effective nerve calming herb. Drink a fresh cup as needed.

Other important herbs are St. John's wort and passion flower. Look for formulas containing all herbs specific for stress.

Vitamins and Minerals

- **B complex**—known as the "stress" vitamins, they are needed for energy and to supply essential cofactors for the nervous system. Take a 50 mg complex twice daily.
- ○ **High potency multi-vitamin without iron**—take on a daily basis for general support.
- ○ **Vitamin C with bioflavonoids**—stored in high concentration in the adrenal glands for the formation of stress hormones. Take 1,000 mg twice daily.
- ○ **Zinc**—there is an increased need for this mineral when stress levels are high. Take 30 mg **with** 3 mg of **copper** with meals.

Other

- **Exercise**—daily exercise reduces stress.
- **Mental imagery**—imagine a relaxing scene. Consider t'ai chi and yoga as forms of stress reduction.
- ○ **Homeopathic *Kali phos* 6x**—take a dose three times daily to help the nervous system cope with stress.
- ○ **Homeopathic Rescue Remedy**—an effective homeopathic combination that helps relax the nervous system. Take as directed on the container.
- ○ Consider **acupuncture** from a qualified practitioner.
- ○ Consider **counseling** for stress coping techniques.

TMJ Syndrome

Temporomandibular Joint Syndrome is a dysfunction of the area where the jaw (mandible) connects to the side of the head (temporal area). Common symptoms include jaw and ear pain; muscle spasms of the facial muscles; difficulty opening the jaw; grinding, clicking and popping of the jaw; and headaches. There can be a number of underlying causes including stress (which tightens muscles and pulls jaw joints out of alignment), improper bite, spinal misalignment and previous trauma to the area. Many cases can be treated without surgery which should be a last resort.

Nutrition

○ While in an **acute state eat soups** for minimal chewing.
○ **Avoid** foods that require **excessive chewing** such as gum, and foods that are hard to chew.
○ Cut **food into small pieces** so that a wide bite is not required.

Herbal

○ **Valerian**—an antispasmodic. Take 1 capsule (150 mg) or 30 drops three times daily. Take more often for acute flare-ups.
○ **Kava kava**—an antispasmodic. Take 1 capsule or 30 drops three times daily. Take more often for acute flare-ups.
○ **Chamomile tea**—relaxes the nervous system. Drink a fresh cup as needed.

Consider also herbs found in *Stress* section.

Vitamins and Minerals

○ **B complex**—helps the body deal with stress. Take a 50 mg complex daily.
○ **Calcium**—relaxes muscles. Take 1,000 mg in divided doses daily.
○ **Magnesium**—relaxes the muscles. Take 500 mg twice daily.
○ **Vitamin C with bioflavonoids**—repairs connective tissue. Take 1,000 mg three times daily.

Other

● Consider **acupuncture** from a qualified practitioner.
● Consider **massage therapy** from a qualified practitioner.
● Consider a **dentist who specializes in TMJ** problems.
● Consider **spinal manipulation** or **chiropractic**.

- Consider **craniosacral therapy** from a qualified practitioner.
- ○ Homeopathic *Mag phos* **6x**—relaxes muscle tissue. Take a dose three times daily.
- ○ Homeopathic *Kali Phos* **6x**—reduces stress and relaxes nerves. Take a dose three times daily.
- ○ Consider **biofeedback training**.

Ulcers

The term ulcer generally refers to erosions in the stomach and more commonly in the duodenum (first part of the small intestine). Pain is often experienced half an hour to an hour after a meal. The *Heliobacter pylori* bacteria has been implicated as a causative agent in symptomatic ulcer patients. Antacids usually provide temporary relief. I recommend removing the causes of the digestive inflammation and simultaneously using natural medicines known to heal the stomach and duodenal mucosa lining. A proper diagnosis is important because bleeding ulcers can be life threatening.

Nutrition

- Identify and eliminate **food allergies** and **sensitivities** as they promote ulcer formation (see *Appendix E*).
- **Avoid** the following as they exacerbate this condition: caffeine, alcohol, refined sugar, tobacco and aspirin.
- ○ **Avoid milk** as long-term use can actually increase stomach acid. Use **milk alternatives** such as rice milk or soy milk.
- ○ **Increase fiber** intake as it helps neutralize acid. Add high fiber foods to the diet such as apples, oat bran, broccoli, Brussels sprouts, cabbage, carrots, wholegrain flour and green leafy vegetables.
- ○ If needed, take a **fiber supplement** composed of psyllium seed husks. Take 2 to 3 capsules daily with eight ounces of purified water.
- ○ **Fresh vegetable juices** containing **cabbage** and **aloe vera** juice are recommended as they promote ulcer healing.

Herbal

The following herbs heal the digestive tract. They should be taken for a minimum of two months:

- **Slippery elm**—take 1 capsule or 30 drops three times daily.
- **Licorice root**—heals the lining of the stomach and intestine. Take 1,000 to 1,500 mg of **deglycyrrhizinated** licorice root or 30 drops of extract three times daily on an empty stomach.
- **Chamomile**—take 1 capsule, 30 drops or 1 cup of tea three times daily.
- ○ **Cat's claw** (3% alkaloids)—heals the digestive tract and eliminates infections in the gastrointestinal tract. Take 1 capsule (200 mg) three times daily.
- ○ **Geranium**—take 1 capsule or 30 drops three times daily.
- ○ **Peppermint**—take 1 capsule, 10 drops or 1 cup of tea three times daily.

Vitamins and Minerals

- **Zinc**—needed to build the stomach's protective lining. Take 30 to 50 mg daily **with** 3 to 5 mg of **copper** with meals.
- **Glutamine**—accelerates healing of ulcers. Take 500 mg three times daily.
- ○ **B complex**—repairs the gastrointestinal tract. Take a 50 mg B complex daily.
- ○ **Quercitin**—decreases histamine response in the stomach and thereby decreases inflammation. Take 500 mg three times daily.
- ○ **Vitamin E**—a natural anti-inflammatory. Take 800 IU daily with a meal.
- ○ **Vitamin A**—heals the stomach and intestinal mucosa. Take 50,000 IU daily for one month.

Other

- **Stress reduction** techniques—such as exercise, mental imagery, counseling and others.

- Constitutional hydrotherapy—see *Appendix A*.
- Homeopathic *Nux vomica* 30C—useful for acute relief of ulcer pain and healing. Take a dose twice daily.
- Homeopathic *Nat phos* 6x—neutralizes excess acidity. Take a dose three times daily between meals.
- Acidophilus—increases beneficial bacteria in the digestive tract. Take as directed on container.
- Consider homeopathy or Chinese herbal medicine from a qualified practitioner.
- Avoid smoking as it prevents healing.

Urinary Tract Infection

Urinary tract (bladder and urethra) infections are generally caused by the *Escherichia coli* bacteria. Common symptoms include burning on urination, a sense of urgency to urinate, fever and fatigue. Complications can occur when the infection ascends to the kidneys—this is serious and requires a physician's supervision. Chronic infections can be due to food allergies and sensitivities. Identifying and removing the offending foods can be very effective for prevention of this condition. Also, females should avoid wiping from the anus to the vagina since feces contain the *E. coli* bacteria. Hormonal imbalances may cause urinary tract infections in women. Sexually transmitted diseases can also present similar symptoms and must be ruled out by a physician.

Nutrition

- Identify and eliminate food allergies and sensitivities (see *Appendix E*).
- Drink eight to ten glasses of purified water daily to flush out germs.
- Avoid the following foods which can aggravate or promote this condition: sugar products and acidic foods such as citrus fruits (orange, lime, lemon, grapefruit) and tomatoes.
- Unsweetened cranberry juice—a natural urinary antiseptic. Drink four to six glasses daily.

Herbal

- **Horsetail**—specific for fighting urinary system infections. Take 2 capsules or 60 drops every two hours until symptoms subside.
- **Echinacea**—stimulates the immune system. Take 2 capsules or 60 drops every two hours.
- **Goldenseal**—antibacterial and stimulates the immune system. Take 2 capsules or 60 drops every two hours.
- ○ **Chimaphila**—specific for fighting urinary system infections. Take 2 capsules or 60 drops every two to three hours until symptoms subside.
- ○ **Marshmallow root**—soothes an irritated urinary tract. Take 2 capsules or 60 drops every two to three hours.
- ○ **Cranberry capsules** (18:1)—an antiseptic for the urinary tract. Take 500 mg four times daily.
- ○ **Uva ursi** (10% arbutin)—antiseptic to the urinary tract. Take 2 capsules or 60 drops every two hours until improvement.

Vitamins and Minerals

- ○ **Vitamin C with bioflavonoids**—take 1,000 mg three to four times daily.

Other

- **Constitutional hydrotherapy**—see *Appendix A*.
- **Homeopathic *Cantharis* 30C**—eliminates urinary tract infections when burning occurs with urination. Take a dose three times daily until condition resolves.
- ○ **Acidophilus**—replenishes the beneficial bacteria of the urinary tract. It is common for an imbalance to occur after antibiotic use. Take 2 capsules twice daily for two months.
- ○ Consider **homeopathy** from a qualified practitioner.
- ○ Consider **acupuncture** and **Chinese herbal medicine** from a qualified practitioner.

Varicose Veins

This condition is characterized by dilated superficial veins and is most common in the legs. When the veins' valves do not work properly blood pools in the vessels resulting in bulging, stretched veins. Some conditions that cause a predisposition to varicose veins include nutritional deficiencies, prolonged sitting or standing in one spot, overweight and lack of exer cise. Aches and pains often accompany the bluish-purple discoloration of the leg veins.

Nutrition

○ Eat a **high fiber diet** with grains.

○ If dietary changes are difficult, take a **fiber supplement** composed of psyllium seed husks. Take 1 to 2 capsules twice daily with an eight ounce glass of purified water.

○ Eat fruit that contains substances for blood vessel health such as **cherries, blueberries** and **blackberries**.

○ Eat **garlic, onions** and **ginger** liberally.

○ **Increase water intake**—drink six to eight glasses of purified water daily.

Herbal

The following herbs are all known for their ability to tonify and reduce swelling of varicose veins:

● **Witch hazel tincture**—apply topically on veins twice daily.

● **Hawthorn berry** (1.8% vitexin-4'rhamnoside)—take 250 mg or 30 drops three times daily.

● **Horse chestnut**—take 1 capsule or 30 drops three times daily.

○ **Butcher's broom** (10% ruscogenin)—1 capsule (300 mg) or 30 drops three times daily.

○ **Bilberry** (25% anthocyanosides)—take 80 mg three times daily.

○ **Gingko** (24% standardized extract)—take 1 capsule or 30 drops three times daily.

Vitamins and Minerals

● **Grape seed extract (PCO)**—take 1 capsule (50 mg) three times daily with meals.

○ **Vitamin C with bioflavonoids**—take 1,000 mg three times daily.

○ **Vitamin E**—reduces inflammation of the blood vessels. Take 800 IU daily with a meal.

○ **Coenzyme Q10**—an antioxidant that improves circulation through the vessels and prevents free radical damage. Take 30 mg three times daily.

○ **Magnesium**—promotes blood vessel health. Take 500 mg daily.

○ **Bromelain**—anti-inflammatory. Take 500 mg three times daily.

Other

● **Foot hydrotherapy**—see *Appendix A*.

● **Exercise**—aerobic exercise (swimming, walking, aerobics) for a minimum of half an hour three to six times weekly. Avoid prolonged standing.

● **Homeopathic *Hammamelis* 6C**—take a dose three times daily for two months.

○ **Constitutional hydrotherapy**—see *Appendix A*.

○ **Homeopathic *Calc fluor* 6x**—take a dose three times daily.

○ Use **elastic stockings**. Women can use pantihose for support of blood vessels.

○ Consider **Chinese herbal medicine** from a qualified practitioner.

Warts

These skin lesions are caused by a virus known as HPV. They are most commonly found on the hands, fingers, forearms, knees, face, feet and genital area (genital warts). Common warts are not usually painful. By enhancing the immune system one can eliminate the HPV virus and thus the wart growths.

Nutrition

○ **Avoid refined sugars**.

○ Eat plenty of **fruits** and **vegetables**.

Herbal

● **Thuja oil**—apply a few drops to wart(s) twice daily.

○ **Echinacea** (4% echinacosides and 0.7% flavonoids)—stimulates the immune system and is antiviral. Take 2 capsules (250 mg) or 30 drops twice daily.

○ **Flaxseed oil**—used for skin eruptions. Take 2 capsules three times daily or 1 tablespoon oil daily.

○ **Lomatium root**—stimulates the immune system to fight viruses. Take 30 drops of extract three times daily.

○ **Garlic**—is antiviral. Take standardized extract daily containing 4,000 mcg allicin.

Vitamins and Minerals

The following vitamins enhance immune system function and eliminate the virus that causes warts:

● **Beta-carotene**—take 100,000 IU daily.

● **Vitamin E**—take 400 IU daily.

● **Vitamin C with bioflavonoids**—take 1,000 mg three to four times daily.

● **Zinc**—take 30 mg daily **with** 3 mg of **copper**.

○ **Vitamin A**—take 10,000 mg daily.

Other

● Consider **homeopathy** from a qualified practitioner.

○ **Hypnosis** has been a good therapy for eliminating warts.

○ Consider **acupuncture** and **Chinese herbal medicine** from a qualified practitioner.

○ **Tape a piece of banana peel to the wart**. Change daily and continue for one month. This treatment is often used for warts on the feet.

○ **Salmon oil**—supplies omega-3 fatty acids for skin health. Take 2 capsules (1,000 mg each) twice daily.

Weight Loss

Weight loss is a misunderstood health topic as is the fallacy of an "ideal" body weight. In general, a body fat percentage above 30% for women and 25% for men is medically termed obesity. It is well known that extra body weight increases the risk for conditions such as diabetes and heart disease. Common sense and patience is needed when preparing a guideline for weight loss. Rapid weight loss programs almost always lead to a rebound phenomenon whereby weight is quickly lost but then gained back along with additional pounds. There are many reasons why people are overweight. These include:

1. **Dietary causes:**
   * High percentage of saturated fat in the diet—saturated fat is the harmful fat found in animal and dairy products and that can lead to weight gain.
   * High intake of refined sugars—the body converts excess sugar into fat.
   * Imbalance between complex carbohydrates and protein intake—excessive carbohydrate consumption can lead to weight gain for some. Those susceptible to this type of reaction will lose weight on a diet that is evenly balanced between carbohydrates and protein.
   * Lack of fiber in the diet—when fiber is consumed with a meal it binds the fats thereby preventing excess fat from being absorbed through the intestines. Fiber is contained in many vegetables (such as leafy green vegetables, broccoli, cauliflower) and fruits with fibrous covering (such as apples).
   * Food Allergies and Sensitivities—frequent consumption of food allergens leads to water retention.

2. **Lack of exercise**. Exercise "burns off" excess calories and fat, and more importantly increases basal body metabolism over time.

3. **Biochemical imbalances.** Hormones and neurotransmitters are very powerful chemicals in the body. Imbalances in these endogenous chemicals may need to be corrected before weight loss can occur. A classic example is women who suffer from low thyroid function after childbirth. Until the thyroid hormone levels are elevated weight loss is very difficult.

4. **Mental and emotional blockages.** Psychological blockages can prevent loss of excess weight. A history of emotional trauma can be the underlying cause of weight gain.

Nutrition

○ In general, consume a diet that follows these guidelines:

- **low in saturated fats**—such as red meat and dairy products
- **low in refined sugars**
- **medium amounts of complex carbohydrates**
- **medium amounts of protein**—fish, legumes, skinless turkey or chicken breast, tofu, nuts
- **high in fiber**—helps to eliminate fats through the digestive system and gives a sense of fullness when eating. High fiber foods include oat bran, green leafy vegetables, broccoli, apples, Brussels sprouts, carrots and whole grains.

○ If needed take a **fiber supplement** that has psyllium seed husks as the base of the formula. Drink at least eight ounces of purified water with each dose.

○ Eat **smaller, more frequent meals** throughout the day, do not skip breakfast. This will prevent the blood sugar levels from jumping up and down which leads to increased insulin levels and fat storage.

○ **Avoid eating out**.

○ **Avoid** alcohol, artificial sweeteners, commercial fat substitutes and caffeine products.

○ **Increase water intake**—drink at least six to eight glasses of purified water daily for proper detoxification and metabolism.

○ **Fresh fruit** and **vegetable juices** are an excellent source of essential nutrients with low calorie and fat content. They also promote excretion of excess water out of the body.

○ Try the **Natural Physician Detox Juicing Recipe** daily for one month: five medium-sized carrots, apple, burdock root (half portion), half a celery stick.

○ Identify and **eliminate food allergies** and **sensitivities** (see *Appendix E*), they interfere with metabolism and cause weight gain due to water retention.

Herbal

○ **Hydroxycitric acid (HCA)**—stimulates metabolism of fat cells and decreases hunger. Take as directed on container.

○ **Flaxseed oil**—supplies essential fatty acids necessary for fat metabolism. Take 1 tablespoon daily.

○ **Dandelion root**—works to improve liver and gall-bladder function which helps in digesting fats. Take 1 capsule or 30 drops before each meal for one to two months.

○ **Plant enzymes**—help digest and assimilate food efficiently. Take with meals as directed on container.

Vitamins and Minerals

The following vitamins are used in fat metabolism and a deficiency of these may impair weight loss:

● **Chromium**—used by the body to utilize blood sugar properly and thus promotes lean muscle mass. Take 200 mcg daily.

○ **L-Carnitine**—provides a cofactor necessary for fat metabolism. Take 500 mg daily.

○ **High potency multi-vitamin without iron**—take daily to ensure against nutritional deficiencies.

○ **B complex**—helps to metabolize carbohydrates efficiently. Take a 50 mg complex daily.

○ **Magnesium**—a deficiency of this mineral can contribute to sweet cravings. Take 250 mg twice daily.

Other

○ Consider **hypnosis** from a qualified practitioner.

○ **Exercise regularly**. Do aerobic exercise three to five times weekly for a minimum of half an hour.

○ **Counseling**—explore mental/emotional obstacles.

○ **Thyroid activity**—have your physician check for thyroid dysfunction as it controls metabolism.

○ **Thyroid glandular**—use if the thyroid gland is underactive. Take 1 tablet three times daily until metabolism increases.

Yeast Infection (Vaginitis)

Candida albicans can be a normal inhabitant of the vagina but overgrowth of this yeast can lead to infection and the following symptoms: itching, burning, odor, and thick, white discharge. Chronic infections are often caused by food sensitivities. Hormonal imbalance can also lead to chronic infections since the pH of the vaginal tissue is highly influenced by hormones such as estrogen, progesterone and testosterone. Long-term use of oral contraceptives and antibiotics can wipe out beneficial bacteria from the vagina and lead to chronic infections.

Nutrition

● Eliminate common allergens such as dairy, wheat, citrus fruit and peanuts from the diet to see if the condition improves. See **Elimination and Reintroduction Diet**—*Appendix E.*

○ **Avoid** refined sugar products, alcohol, caffeine and tobacco products.

○ Eat **plain yogurt** as it contains beneficial bacteria for the vagina.

Herbal

● **Goldenseal**—immune stimulant. Take 2 capsules or 30 drops three to four times daily.

○ **Garlic**—antiviral, antibacterial and antifungal. Take 2 capsules 4,000 mcg of standardized allicin content extract twice daily.

○ **Echinacea** (4% echinacosides and 0.7% flavonoids)—an immune system stimulant. Take 2 capsules (250 mg each) or 30 drops three to four times daily.

○ **Calendula douche**—useful for acute yeast infections. Put 60 drops of calendula extract in glass of water and apply as a douche into the vagina. Repeat once daily for five days.

Vitamins and Minerals

The following vitamins enhance the immune system function to help fight the vaginal infection:

● **Vitamin C with bioflavonoids**—take 1,000 mg three times daily.

○ **Beta-carotene**—take 100,000 IU daily.

○ **Zinc**—immune stimulant. Take 30 mg daily.

○ **Copper**—works in conjunction with **zinc**. Take 3 mg daily.

○ **High potency multi-vitamin without iron**—take daily to correct any nutritional deficiencies.

Other

● **Acidophilus**—take 2 capsules three times daily or as directed on container. As well, insert one capsule into the vagina and cover with a pad. This should be done morning and evening.

● **Boric acid**—for yeast infections, insert a capsule into the vagina and cover with a pad. This should be done morning and evening for up to fourteen days.

○ **Wear cotton underwear** to prevent moisture build-up.

○ **Plain yogurt**—apply to vaginal area. It provides beneficial bacteria which help to destroy infections and rebalance the flora.

○ **Homeopathy** from a qualified practitioner.

○ **Chinese herbal medicine** from a qualified practitioner.

APPENDIX A

Natural Physician Hydrotherapy Guide

Hydrotherapy refers to the therapeutic use of water (internally or externally) for the prevention and treatment of illness. Water can be used in many different forms such as hot, cold, steam, ice and applied to the body through various techniques such as whirlpools, towels, wraps, poultices, fomentations and colonic irrigations. The following characteristics of water are utilized through hydrotherapy:

- water absorbs and transfers large amounts of heat and cold
- due to its fluidity water is easily applied to the skin and body contours

Hydrotherapy is a simple but very effective technique to optimize the circulation of blood and lymph. For example, short-term use of heat stimulates and dilates the blood vessels which in turn increases tissue oxygenation and the excretion of tissue waste products. The use of cold over a short period of time increases white blood cell count and also increases tissue oxygenation and waste excretion.

Circulation can be manipulated in the body for therapeutic effects. For example, headaches can be relieved by putting the feet in warm water and placing an ice pack around the neck. The warm water dilates the blood vessels in the feet, increases blood flow to the feet and moves the congested blood from the head. As well, the ice pack constricts the blood vessels in the neck and head area which reduces congestion.

Hydrotherapy treatments can be applied over a large body surface for general tonification, as in cancer treatment. Cancer can be viewed as a systemic breakdown of the immune system, and hydrotherapy applied to large areas of the body stimulates of the immune system. Local applications   such as the foot hydrotherapy can be used to focus on specific problem areas.

Hydrotherapy is also used to enhance a fever reaction in the body since proper application of hot and cold evokes an immune response. This can be useful for many conditions since fever stimulates the immune system. By working with a fever, toxins and infections are eliminated more effectively.

Detoxification is another benefit of hydrotherapy. Enhancement of circulation through the eliminatory organs such as the liver, kidneys, digestive tract and skin removes toxins and improves blood quality.

History of Hydrotherapy

Naturopathic hydrotherapy was developed by a line of brilliant health practitioners. One of the first was Vincent Priessnitz (1799–1852). As a farmboy in Austria, he noticed how injured animals instinctively bathed their injuries in cold water. He applied this observation by using hydrotherapy to speed the healing process for his own farm animals. At the age of seventeen he broke two ribs. The local surgeon could not help him so Priessnitz reduced the fracture himself and quickly recovered by applying hydrotherapy to his chest. He then went on to treat thousands of people with diet and hydrotherapy treatments.

Another notable hydrotherapist was Father Sebastian Kneipp (1821–1897). He was initially rejected from the priesthood because he suffered from tuberculosis. He cured himself of this disease with hydrotherapy and diet and began using these same treatments on parishioners. Many thousands of people were relieved of their illness through his hydrotherapy treatments.

Followers of Priessnitz and Kneipp brought the practice of hydrotherapy to North America. Benedict Lust (1872–1945), known as the "Father of Naturopathy," greatly influenced the promotion of hydrotherapy and naturopathic medicine in the United States. While a young German immigrant living in the U.S., Lust developed a life threatening case of tuberculosis—medical doctors gave him no chance of recovery. In a last attempt to save his life Benedict Lust traveled to Germany for treatments by Father Kneipp. Lust completely regained his health and returned to the United States to practice and spread the hydrotherapy techniques of Father Kneipp.

Conventional medicine also has a lineage of hydrotherapy practitioners. John Harvey Kellogg (1852–1943), founder of the Kellogg's cereal company, was a medical doctor who used hydrotherapy as a primary treatment at his Battle Creek clinic in Michigan.

Hydrotherapy continued its evolution and passage to become a treatment method of modern naturopaths. It is taught in naturopathic medical schools across North America and in Europe. This appendix describes three different hydrotherapy treatments that can be done at home: constitutional hydrotherapy with an assistant, constitutional hydrotherapy without an assistant and foot hydrotherapy.

Constitutional Hydrotherapy
This treatment has been perfected by naturopathic doctors over the past fifty years. It can be conveniently done in the comfort of home with or without an assistant. When used properly it accomplishes five major goals:

- optimizes circulation
- detoxifies and purifies the blood
- enhances digestive function and elimination
- tonifies and balances the nervous system
- stimulates and enhances the immune system

Conditions commonly treated include:

- *Digestive problems:* Crohn's disease, irritable bowel syndrome, peptic ulcer, ulcerative colitis, constipation, diarrhea, heartburn
- *Respiratory problems:* asthma, bronchitis, pneumonia, sore throat
- *Infections:* colds, flus, bladder infection, ear infection
- *Immune system deficiency:* cancer, allergies, chronic fatigue syndrome
- *Circulatory problems:* Raynaud's disease, varicose veins, hypertension, hemorrhoids
- *Inflammatory problems:* arthritis, psoriasis, lupus, multiple sclerosis
- *Female problems:* PMS, menstrual cramps, infertility
- *Male problems:* prostate enlargement, prostatitis, impotence

Frequency:

- *Chronic conditions:* three to five treatments weekly
- *Acute conditions:* once or twice daily

Directions—With an Assistant:

1. Patient lies flat on back.
2. Cover the bared chest and abdomen with two thickness of towel that have been placed in hot water then wrung out (wet towels can also be heated in a microwave). Towels should be as hot as patient can comfortably tolerate.
3. Cover the body with two large blankets to avoid chilling. Rest for five minutes.
4. After five minutes remove the hot towels and replace with a single thickness of a thin towel that has been run under cold water and then wrung out (leave some moisture in the towel).
5. Place the cold towel on the bared chest and abdomen and put the blankets back on. Do not place hot towels back on cold towels.
6. Leave the cold towel in place for ten minutes or longer until it becomes warmed (usually ten to fifteen minutes).
7. Have person turn over and lay on their abdomen. Repeat the same procedure on the back.

Directions—Without an Assistant:

1. Take a hot bath or shower for five minutes.
2. Get out and dry yourself quickly.
3. Place a towel in cold water then wring it out and wrap it around your trunk (from armpits to groin).
4. Cover with a blanket (preferably wool) to avoid chilling.
5. Leave the cold towel in place for at least twenty minutes, or longer, until it is warmed.

Foot Hydrotherapy

This treatment is used for different conditions than the constitutional hydrotherapy. The treatment focuses the blood flow towards the feet thus reducing upper body congestion.

Conditions commonly treated include:

- sinusitis, respiratory congestion, pelvic congestion, headaches, nosebleed and other upper body conditions
- good for insomnia as it promotes relaxation

Frequency:

- *Chronic conditions:* three to five treatments weekly until condition resolved
- *Acute conditions:* once or twice daily

Directions:

1. Soak both feet in a bucket of warm water (as hot as can be tolerated) for five to ten minutes.
2. Remove feet from water and dry them.
3. Put on a pair of cotton socks that have been placed in cold water and wrung out.
4. Cover with another pair of socks (preferably wool).
5. Rest for half an hour or more. It is best to leave the socks on until they are dry.

APPENDIX B

Natural Physician Homeopathy Guide

Homeopathy is a complete system of medicine based on the premise that "like cures like." In other words, a substance that can produce symptoms in a healthy person can also be used to treat an ill person who has those same symptoms. This is similar to the concept of vaccines, whereby a minute amount of a disease-causing agent is used to stimulate the protective and healing properties of the immune system. Homeopathics are extremely dilute substances that are generally prepared from plant, mineral and animal sources.

When used for the proper indications they work to:

- stimulate and repair the immune system
- balance mental and emotional states
- repair general imbalances in or physical damage to the body

Homeopathy is a very popular system of medicine used all over the world by physicians and health practitioners. It has been estimated that fifty percent of the medical doctors in Germany prescribe homeopathic medicines or refer to practitioners of homeopathy. Homeopathy is very popular in many European countries such as France, Belgium and England. For over a hundred years the Royal Family in England has used the services of medical practitioners that specialize in homeopathy. As well, India has tens of thousands of practitioners that use homeopathy exclusively in their practice.

There are four main reasons why homeopathy is so widely used:

- It is highly effective for chronic and acute diseases, including epidemics. Homeopathy works to strengthen the immune system and can treat viruses and other conditions for which conventional medicine has no effective treatment.
- It is cost effective. Compared to pharmaceutical medications, homeopathic medicines are quite inexpensive.
- It is a preventative medicine. One does not have to have a disease to be treated with homeopathy. It can be used to optimize health.

- It *treats the whole person*. Homeopathy takes into account all the factors of a person's health—the mental, emotional and physical.

History of Homeopathy

Homeopathy and its principles can be traced back to ancient medical texts dating back as far as 1,000 B.C. The famous Greek physician Hippocrates made reference to the principles of homeopathy in his medical writings. The most prominent figure in the roots and development of homeopathy was Samuel Hahnemann (1755–1845), a German physician and scholar. Dr. Hahnemann abandoned his medical practice after becoming disillusioned with crude and barbaric treatments such as bloodletting, purging and using lethal doses of poisonous substances such as mercury and arsenic to treat disease.

Dr. Hahnemann was a brilliant scholar, chemist and scientist and used his talents to pioneer modern homeopathy. It was during his translation of a book on medicinal substances that he came across the concept of homeopathy. The author of the book stated that cinchona bark was able to cure malaria in many cases due to its bitter taste. Hahnemann was not satisfied with this explanation and took the extract of the cinchona bark to experience its effects. After taking successive doses he developed symptoms of sweating, chills, general malaise and weakness—the same symptoms as malaria.

This self-experiment led to the realization (also discovered by other physicians such as Hippocrates) that "like cures like" also known as the law of similars. In other words, substances that cause particular symptoms in healthy persons can stimulate healing in those who are ill with similar symptoms. A simple example of this process is the homeopathic *Apis*, a preparation of bee venom. The common symptoms of a bee sting are stinging, burning, redness and swelling. These are the same symptoms that can be relieved by the homeopathic *Apis*. It does not matter if the symptoms are caused by a bee sting, arthritis or a urinary tract infection. If the symptoms match those of the homeopathic, a cure can occur as the body's healing mechanisms are activated by the law of similars. Hahnemann coined this medical system homeopathy, after the Greek words *homios* which means similar, and *pathos* which means suffer.

Hahnemann and others tested many different substances to determine which symptoms they cause and for what illnesses they may be indicated. After much experimentation Hahnemann found that homeopathics became more effective and had fewer side-effects when prepared by a special process of dilution and succussion (exertion of a shaking or pounding force on the medicines). This process is referred to as potentization and indicates the strength of the homeopathic. Today special laboratory equipment is used in pharmacies throughout the world in the production of homeopathics.

How to Use Homeopathics

Homeopathics are best taken ten to twenty minutes away from food or drink. They are available in pellet, tablet or liquid form. Use as directed on the container or use the following guidelines:

- **Pellet or tablet**—therapeutic ingredients in sucrose pills. *One dose equals 2 pellets or tablets* (for children and adults). Dissolve in mouth.
- **Liquid**—therapeutic ingredients in water and small amounts of alcohol. *One dose equals 10 to 20 drops* (for children and adults). Dissolve in mouth.

Potency refers to the strength of the medicine. The number behind the homeopathic indicates the dilution and the strength of the medicine. The higher the number the stronger the action of the medicine, e.g., *Kali phos* 6x is stronger than *Kali phos* 3x.

These are two main scales of potency used in homeopathy:

- **"x" potency**—these are the lowest potencies used. The first dilution is equal to 1 part of the original substance to 9 parts of solvent.
- **"C" potency**—the first dilution is equal to 1 part of the original substance to 99 parts of solvent.

Use the potencies recommended in the treatment sections of this book. If none is given I recommend the 6x, 6C or 30C potencies.

Repetition refers to how often the homeopathic is repeated. The following guides can be used for adults and children:

- **Acute illness:** take homeopathic as often as is needed for relief of symptoms and recovery from the illness. Emergencies such as hemorrhage may need the medicine repeated every five minutes. Less severe conditions such as a sinus infection may need medicine to be taken twice daily or less. Follow directions given in the treatment sections of this book or repeat until improvement is noticed.

- **Chronic illness:** the lower x or C potencies are often taken once or twice daily until symptoms improve and then used as needed to continue improvement. Follow directions given in the treatment sections of this book.

Natural Physician First Aid Homeopathics

The following homeopathics are commonly needed for acute care. They are prescribed on physical, mental and emotional symptoms.

Aconite *(Aconitum napellus)* monkshood

Symptoms come on very quickly when this medicine is needed. This can be a fever or beginning of an infection. Exposure to the cold, dry wind may bring on this state. Person exhibits panic, restlessness and fear with the illness. It is also useful for emotional complaints after a sudden shock or fright to calm a person down. This medicine works best when taken in the beginning stage of an illness.

Conditions: cold, fever, sore throat, ear infection, panic disorder, bladder infection

Apis *(Apis mellifica)* honey-bee

Used for illness with symptoms similar to a bee sting such as stinging, burning, redness and swelling. This can range from the reaction from a bee sting to a sore throat. The application of warmth or pressure makes the symptoms worse but relief is had by cool applications or open air. Thirst is usually low.

Conditions: bee sting, arthritis, bladder or kidney infection, herpes, ovarian cyst, sore throat, shingles

Arnica *(Arnica montana)* leopard's bane

An excellent medicine for physical trauma. It is the first homeopathic given after an injury or trauma. This can range from strained ligaments to bruised muscles. People benefiting from arnica typically have a bruised sensation with the injury. It is beneficial for shock associated with an injury, particularly when the person feels they do not need medical attention but have sustained a trauma.

Conditions: bruises, concussion, sprains, strains, post surgical recovery, hemorrhage, labor

Arsenicum *(Arsenicum album)* arsenic trioxide

Symptoms that are present for this medicine include anxiety, restlessness, weakness and exhaustion, chilliness and burning pains. Symptoms are often worse between midnight to 3 A.M. and are aggravated by cold air and improved with warm applications. Mental symptoms of great fear and anxiety are often present.

Conditions: allergies, anxiety, asthma, cancer, colds, depression, diarrhea, flu, food poisoning, herpes, ulcer, urinary tract infection, vomiting

Belladonna *(Atropa belladonna)* deadly nightshade

Useful for inflammatory conditions. Presenting symptoms are high fever, dilated pupils, throbbing pain, worse being moved or jarred, and a flushed face. Person may have hallucinations due to the high fever. Thirst is usually low.

Conditions: boils, febrile convulsions, painful menses, ear infections, throat infection, migraine headache, ovarian pain

Bryonia *(Bryonia alba)* wild hop, white bryony

Useful homeopathic for acute disorders, especially of the mucous membranes and musculoskeletal system. Symptoms include aggravation from motion (desire to be completely still), irritability, dryness, great thirst and left-sided complaints.

Conditions: appendicitis, arthritis, bronchitis, cough, flu, mastitis, migraine, headache, pleurisy, pneumonia, sprains, strains, tendinitis

Cantharis *(Cantharis vesicator)* Spanish fly

Important homeopathic for burns and conditions that bring on burning pains.

Conditions: burns, bladder and kidney infections

Chamomile *(Matricaria chamomilla)*
This medicine is indicated when there is hypersensitivity to pain. Person is very irritable and inconsolable. Children in this state are worse with warmth and lying down. They feel better while carried and rocked.
Conditions: colic, earache, teething, tooth pain (general)

Ferrum phos *(Ferrum phosphoricum)* phosphate of iron
Useful in the first stages of an inflammatory condition. Presenting symptoms are fever, flushed face and fatigue. Person may not act sick with these symptoms. Also, useful for bleeding or hemorrhage.
Conditions: anemia, bursitis, bleeding (general), bleeding nose, cold, flu, ear infection, sore throat

Gelsemium *(Gelsemium sempervirens)* yellow jasmine
Physical and mental weakness are the main symptoms with this medicine. The body can feel tired and weary, the limbs may feel heavy. There can be muscle aching and stiffness and chills that run through the body. Person is thirstless. The person becomes drowsy, forgetful and weary. They may experience diarrhea from anxiety.
Conditions: chronic fatigue immunodeficiency syndrome, diarrhea, flu, headache, multiple sclerosis, tremor, vertigo

Hepar sulph *(Hepar sulphuris calcareum)* sulphide of calcium
Person is hypersensitive to pain and very irritable. They are aggravated by touch, cold, drafts and feel better with warmth and lying on the painless side. Useful in short-term conditions like the flu.
Conditions: abscess, bronchitis, ear/throat infections, flu

Hypericum *(Hypericum perforatum)* St. John's wort
An excellent medicine for trauma to the nerves and spine. A strong symptom is sharp, shooting pains across affected parts of the body.
Conditions: nerve injuries, spinal trauma, lacerations

Ignatia *(Ignatia amara)* St. Ignatius bean
An excellent medicine for acute emotional stress. Patients

that benefit from this medicine have experienced an emotional upset such as grief, anger or disappointment. Person feels like crying alone and is worse with consolation and can have mood swings. The muscles often tense up especially in the neck and shoulder area. There is a lot of sighing and the sensation of a lump in the throat.

Conditions: chorea, depression, mood swings, headache, hysteria, spasms

Ipecac *(Cephaelis ipecacuanha)*

Specific medicine for nausea and vomiting, especially when the nausea does not seemed to be relieved by vomiting. Also used for uterine hemorrhage with nausea, as well as respiratory conditions.

Conditions: asthma, bronchitis, flu, gastroenteritis, hemorrhage, uterine bleeding, migraine headache, morning sickness

Kali bich *(Kali bichromium)* bichromate of potassium

Homeopathic that is indicated when thick, gluey, yellow or green discharges from the mucous membranes are present. Most often indicated for sinus infections.

Conditions: asthma, bronchitis, sinusitis, throat infection

Ledum *(Ledum palustre)* marsh tea, Labrador tea

Specific medicine for the healing of puncture wounds. Also used for animal and insect bites. Wound feels better with cold applications.

Conditions: bites, bruises, puncture wounds, wound infections

Lycopodium *(Lycopodium clavatum)* club moss

This medicine covers a wide range of conditions. It is beneficial for many conditions which affect the digestive system such as flatulence. Persons that benefit from this medicine often have right-sided symptoms, worse 4 P.M. to 8 P.M., crave sweets and are chilly. They are ameliorated from warm applications and warm drinks.

Conditions: asthma, bronchitis, digestive problems, ear infection, headache, sinusitis, urinary tract infection, warts

Mercury *(Mercurius solubilis* and *Mercurius vivus)* quicksilver
Useful medicine for acute conditions where there is
inflammation of the mucous membranes and skin. Person
will have heavy perspiration that does not relieve symptoms,
intolerant to hot and cold temperatures, foul breath,
perspiration and increased salivation.
Conditions: abscess, colds, conjunctivitis, gastroenteritis,
ear infection, sinusitis, throat infection

Nux vomica *(Strychnos nux vomica)* poison-nut
An excellent medicine for the digestive and nervous system.
Patient is chilly, irritable and impatient.
Conditions: alcoholism, asthma, colds, digestive problems
(constipation, stomach cramps, vomiting), flu, headaches

Phosphorus *(Phosphorus)*
This medicine is useful for the respiratory, digestive and
vascular systems. Persons benefiting from this medicine
have a great thirst for cold drinks and are chilly.
Conditions: asthma, bronchitis, cough, fatigue,
hemorrhage, nosebleed, pneumonia, ulcer

Pulsatilla *(Pulsatilla pratensis)* windflower
A very common medicine for acute illnesses. Symptoms
include low thirst, aggravation from heat, changeable
symptoms and amelioration of symptoms from being
consoled or having company. Beneficial for acute conditions
affecting the respiratory and hormonal systems.
Conditions: bronchitis, conjunctivitis, cough, ear infection,
menstrual cramps, sinusitis, throat infection

Rhus tox *(Rhus toxicodredon)* poison ivy, poison oak
Excellent homeopathic for the muscle and joint tissue.
Characteristic symptoms include aching joints and muscles
that are worse at rest and initial movement, but improve
with continued motion. Stiffness and restlessness are strong
symptoms. The pain is worse in cold, damp weather and
symptoms are better with warmth and warm applications.
This medicine is also useful for certain skin rashes.
Conditions: arthritis, herpes, rashes, shingles, sprains

Sulphur (*Sulphur*) brimstone

Useful medicine for skin eruptions and problems with the digestive tract. Skin rashes are very itchy and worse with warmth. Persons benefited by sulphur are often warm, perspire easily and feel better in the open air. They crave spicy foods and have a great thirst for cold drinks.

Conditions: conjunctivitis, eczema, digestive problems (flatulence), skin rashes

Symphytum (*Symphytum officinale*) comfrey

A specific medicine for fractured bones.

Conditions: fractures, tailbone contusion

Schussler Cell Salts (Biochemical Tissue Salts)

This is a simplified but effective system of homeopathy which I recommend for beginners. These homeopathics were researched and developed by Dr. Schussler of Germany. He found that twelve inorganic minerals were key constituents of cells and that a deficiency or imbalance of these cell salts leads to disease. When administered in minute quantities these naturally occurring biochemical tissue cell salts stimulate the cells to assimilate nutrients efficiently. Replenishing and balancing of these minerals restores proper structure and function of each cell, tissue and organ.

How to Use Cell Salts

Cell salt potencies ranges from 1x to 6x with the 3x and 6x potencies most commonly used. These potencies are very safe and side-effects are not an issue. The following are the potencies and amounts I recommend for each age group (*note that these are different dosages than for the other homeopathics*):

- **infants**—1 tablet or 5 drops twice daily
- **children**—2 tablets or 20 drops twice daily
- **adults**—4 to 5 tablets or 20 drops two to three times daily

12 Schussler Cell Salts Summary

Calc fluor (*Calcarea fluorica*) calcium fluoride

Indications: tendon and ligament sprains or tears, bone

tumors, brittle teeth and gums, abnormal spinal curvatures, uterine displacement, hemorrhoids, varicose veins, cataracts

Calc phos *(Calcarea phosphorica)* calcium phosphate
Indications: fractures, teething, growing pains, muscle spasms, osteoporosis

Calc sulph *(Calcarea sulphurica)* gypsum, calcium sulphate
Indications: yellow pus-like discharges from the skin, abscess, boils, acne, ulcers, bronchitis

Ferrum phos *(Ferrum phosphoricum)* ferri phosphate
Indications: cuts, hemorrhage, anemia, nosebleed, sore throat, fever, flu, ear infection

Kali mur *(Kali muriatricum)* potassium chloride
Indications: sore throat, fluid in middle ear

Kali phos *(Kali phosphoricum)* potassium phosphate
Indications: anxiety, nervousness, mental fatigue, nerve injuries or inflammation, chronic fatigue

Kali sulph *(Kali suphuricum)* potassium sulphate
Indications: eczema with yellow discharge, shingles with yellow discharge, psoriasis, ear infection

Mag phos *(Magnesium phosphorica)* magnesium phosphate
Indications: muscle cramps, nerve pain, writer's cramp, painful menses, abdominal cramps, toothache better warm applications

Nat mur *(Natrium muriatricum)* table salt, sodium chloride
Indications: edema, cold sores, migraine, hayfever

Nat phos *(Natrium phosphoricum)* sodium phosphate
Indications: heartburn, muscle soreness, bladder infections, vaginitis

Nat sulph *(Natrium suphuricum)* Glauber's salt, sodium sulphate
Indications: hepatitis, depression, asthma, head injury, warts

Silicea *(Silicea)* quartz, silica
Indications: boil, abscess, pus-like discharges, brittle bones, brittle nails, brittle hair, chronic infections

APPENDIX C

Natural Physician Herbal Medicine Guide

Plants have been used as medicine for thousands of years. It has been estimated by the World Health Organization that close to eighty percent of the world's population use herbal medicine. European medical doctors use herbal medicine routinely in their health care system. As well, over the past fifteen years there has been an explosion in the scientific validation of botanical medicine. Years ago, practitioners of natural medicine relied on folk history and family tradition for therapeutic use of herbal medicine. Today, scientific research has discovered many of the medicinal constituents and verified the uses of common herbal remedies.

Advantages to using herbal medicines over pharmaceutical drugs include:

- fewer side-effects
- less expensive
- treats the cause of illnesses and doesn't just mask the symptoms
- prevents illness
- can often be used for more than one condition since they have a variety of therapeutic effects

How to Use Herbal Medicine

Herbal medicine can be used in the following forms:

Tea: either an infusion—the herb is steeped in hot water (using a tea bag is the most common example); or a decoction—used for more dense plant materials: a half teaspoon of herb per cup of water is boiled for ten to twenty minutes, then let sit until slightly warm. Ginger root is a good example of the type of herb made into a tea by this process.

Capsule: dry herb in a gelatinous capsule

Tincture: (liquid) either preserved in an alcohol solution or a glycerine solution

Compress: liquid extract of a herb that is absorbed across the skin. Take a clean cloth made of cotton, wool, linen or gauze and soak it in a hot infusion or decoction of the prescribed herb(s). While the compress is still warm place it over the affected area. Cover the cloth with plastic or waxed paper. Keep the compress warm (e.g., with a hot water bottle).

Poultice: herb is made into a paste by mixing it with hot water or hot apple cider vinegar. Apply a small amount of olive oil over the skin and then apply the poultice either directly on the skin or between two pieces of thin gauze then onto the affected area. Keep the poultice warm with a hot water bottle or heating pad.

Liniment: preformulated to be absorbed through the skin and applied by massage

Oil: preformulated to be applied topically

Salve: oils or lanolin are used as a base for topical application to form an insulating layer.

Cream: herb is blended with an emulsion of water in oil. Due to the oil component there is a mixing with skin secretions and penetration into the skin.

Standardized Extracts

This refers to the measuring and standardizing of the active ingredients in herbal medicines which guarantees the potency of the herbal product and allows for uniformity in the herbal industry. No plant constituents are withdrawn for the sake of standardization.

There are three types of standardized extracts.

Tincture: herb is soaked in alcohol for a period of time and then pressed and preserved in alcohol and water. The concentration is usually 1:10 or 1:5 (referring to 10 or 5 units of extract from 1 unit of herb).

Fluid extract: a more potent concentration than tinctures. They are made similarly to tinctures but have the alcohol distilled off. The concentration is usually 1:1.

Solid extract: even more potent than fluid extracts. A process similar to fluid extraction is used and then the solvent is completely removed. The extract is then ground into powder or granules. As a potency reference, one gram of a 4:1 solid extract is equivalent to 4 ml of fluid extract or 40 ml of tincture.

Childrens' Dosages
To determine the herbal dosage for a child make the following calculation:

1. Take the adult dose (the dosage listed on bottle or recom mended in the treatment sections of this book) and multiply it by the child's weight.
2. Take this number and divide it by 150.

For example, if the recommended dosage is 60 drops three times daily for an adult and the child is 20 pounds, the two steps would be:

1. 60 x 20 = 1200
2. 1200 ÷ 150 = 8

So 8 drops three times daily would be the child's dosage.

Natural Physician Herbal Medicines
These herbs are used for the treatment of various conditions.

Aloe *(Aloe vera)* Barbados aloe, Curaçao aloe
Medicinal Parts: leaves
Uses: used topically for burns or dry skin, used internally to heal digestive tract, taken internally at moderate dosages as a laxative.

American ginseng *(Panax quinquefolius)*
Medicinal Parts: root
Uses: adaptogen—helps body cope with mental or physical stress, nourishes the adrenal (stress) glands, fatigue

Angelica *(Angelica sinensis)* tang-kuei, dong quai
Medicinal Parts: roots, leaves
Uses: PMS, menopause, painful menses, irregular menses, smooth muscle relaxant, anti-inflammatory, estrogenic effects

Arnica *(Arnica montana)* leopard's bane
Medicinal Parts: flowers, root
Uses: apply oil externally for bruises *(do not use on broken skin)*

Astragalus *(Astragalus membranosus)*
Medicinal Parts: root
Uses: immune stimulant to prevent or treat infections

Bearberry *(Arctostaphylos uva-ursi)* uva-ursi
Medicinal Parts: leaves
Uses: bladder infection, kidney infection, kidney stones

Bilberry *(Vaccinium myrtillus)* huckleberry
Medicinal Parts: leaves, berries
Uses: used to heal connective tissue, cataracts, macular degeneration, diabetic retinopathy, night blindness

Black cohosh *(Cimicifuga racemosa)*
Medicinal Parts: root
Uses: menopause, muscle spasms, depression

Black currant *(Ribies nigrum)* quinsy berry
Medicinal Parts: leaves, fruit
Uses: skin conditions, inflammatory states, bleeding gums

Blue cohosh *(Caulophyllum thalictroides)* squaw root
Medicinal Parts: root
Uses: menstrual cramps, infertility, irregular menses, labor

Burdock *(Arctium lappa)* burr seed
Medicinal Parts: root, seeds
Uses: detoxifies liver and promotes bile flow, purifies the blood, psoriasis, balances hormones

Butcher's broom *(Ruscus aculeatus)*
Medicinal Parts: seeds, tops
Uses: anti-inflammatory, constricts blood vessels, hemorrhoids, varicose veins

Cactus *(Cereus grandiflorus)*
Medicinal Parts: stem, leaves
Uses: heart contraction, congestive heart failure, arrhythmia, circulation

Calendula *(Calendula officinalis)* pot marigold
Medicinal Parts: leaves, flowers
Uses: antiseptic, promotes wound healing, cuts, abrasions

Cascara *(Cascara sagrada)*
Medicinal Parts: bark
Uses: laxative

Cat's claw *(Una de gato)*
Medicinal Parts: root
Uses: anti-inflammatory, immune system enhancement, chronic infections, parasites, ulcers

Cayenne *(Capsicum frutescens)* chili pepper
Medicinal Parts: ripe fruit
Uses: Chills, high cholesterol, circulation, poor digestion, stops bleeding of external cuts, reduces pain

Chamomile *(Matricaria chamomilla)* German chamomile
Medicinal Parts: flowering tops
Uses: anti-inflammatory and antispasmodic for digestive tract, calms nerves, ulcers

Chasteberry *(Vitex agnus castus)* vitex
Medicinal Parts: berry
Uses: menstrual irregularities, cystic ovaries, PMS, menopause

Cherry bark *(Prunus serotina)*
Medicinal Parts: outer and inner barks of stems
Uses: cough

Chionanthus *(Chionanthus virginicus)* fringe tree
Medicinal Parts: bark
Uses: increases bile flow from liver and gall-bladder, jaundice

Cineraria *(Cineraria maritima)* silver ragwort
Medicinal Parts: whole plant
Uses: specific remedy for cataracts

Cinnamon *(Cinnamomum zeylanicum)*
Medicinal Parts: bark, twig
Uses: improves circulation, colds, flus, chills, poor digestion

Collinsonia *(Collinsonia canadensis)* stone root
Medicinal Parts: root
Uses: hemorrhoids, respiratory congestion

Coltsfoot *(Tussilago farfara)* coughwort
Medicinal Parts: leaf, flower
Uses: emphysema, cough, bronchitis

Comfrey *(Symphytum officinale)* knit bone
Medicinal Parts: leaves, roots
Uses: use topically and internally for broken bones, use topically for skin rashes

Cranberry *(Vaccinium macrocarpona)*
Medicinal Parts: fruit
Uses: antiseptic for urinary system, bladder infections

Crampbark *(Viburnum opulus)*
Medicinal Parts: root bark
Uses: antispasmodic for uterus

Dandelion *(Taraxacum officinalis)*
Medicinal Parts: root, leaves
Uses: liver stimulant, diuretic, high blood pressure, PMS

Devil's claw *(Harpagophytum procumbens)*
Medicinal Parts: root
Uses: arthritis, inflammatory conditions

Echinacea *(Echinacea purpurea* or *E. angustifolia)* purple coneflower
Medicinal Parts: root
Uses: any type of infection, colds, a blood purifier

Ephedra *(Lobelia inflata)*
Medicinal Parts: stems, branch, leaves
Uses: respiratory infections, bronchitis, asthma, hayfever

Evening primrose *(Oenothera biennis)*
Medicinal Parts: entire plant
Uses: skin rashes, PMS, multiple sclerosis, inflammatory conditions

Eyebright *(Euphrasia officinalis)*
Medicinal Parts: parts of plant growing above ground
Uses: conjunctivitis, poor eyesight, allergies

Fennel *(Foeniculum vulgare)* sweet fennel
Medicinal Parts: root, seeds
Uses: lung congestion, flatulence, stimulates appetite, poor digestion, hormone balancing

Feverfew *(Tanacetum parthenium)* featherfew
Medicinal Parts: leaves, bark, flowers
Uses: headaches, painful menses

Flax *(Linum usitatissimum)* common flax
Medicinal Parts: seed
Uses: skin disorders, constipation

Garcinia *(Garcinia cambogia)* Hydroxycitric acid (HCA)
Medicinal Parts: fruit
Uses: weight loss

Garlic *(Allium sativum)* clove garlic
Medicinal Parts: bulb
Uses: high blood fats, anti-carcinogenic, lowers blood pressure

Gentian root *(Gentiana lutea)* bitter root
Medicinal Parts: root, rhizome
Uses: low stomach acid, poor digestion, stimulates appetite

Geranium *(Geranium maculatum)*
Medicinal Parts: rhizome
Uses: ulcers, uterine bleeding, diarrhea

Ginger root *(Zingiber officinale)* African ginger
Medicinal Parts: root, rhizome
Uses: flatulence, poor digestion, low appetite, chills

Ginkgo *(Ginkgo biloba)*
Medicinal Parts: leaves
Uses: memory improvement, hearing loss, ringing in ears, Alzheimer's disease, coronary heart disease, poor circulation

Globe artichoke *(Cynara scolymus)* artichoke
Medicinal Parts: flowers, leaves, root
Uses: liver disease, gall-bladder disease

Goldenseal *(Hydrastis canadensis)* yellow root
Medicinal Parts: root
Uses: antibacterial, antiviral, infections, digestion, ulcers

Gotu kola *(Centella asiatica)*
Medicinal Parts: nuts, root, seeds
Uses: memory improvement, detoxifier, connective tissue formation

Gymnemma *(Gymnemma sylvestre)*
Medicinal Parts: leaves
Uses: diabetes

Gugulipid *(Commiphora mukul)*
Medicinal Parts: tree
Uses: lowers triglyceride and cholesterol levels

Hawthorn *(Crataegus oxycantha)* English hawthorn
Medicinal Parts: berries
Uses: high blood pressure, angina, heart disease

Horse chestnut *(Aesculus hippocastanum)* Spanish chestnut
Medicinal Parts: leaves, bark, fruit
Uses: astringent, varicose veins, leg ulcers, hemorrhoids

Horsetail *(Equisetum arvense)*
Medicinal Parts: entire plant
Uses: bladder infection, kidney infection, bed-wetting

Horseradish *(Amoracia lapathifolia)*
Medicinal Parts: root
Uses: sinusitis, diuretic

Kava kava *(Piper methysticum)* kava
Medicinal Parts: rhizome
Uses: anxiety, depression, muscle relaxant, pain

Kelp *(Fucus vesiculosus)* bladderwrack
Medicinal Parts: entire plant
Uses: hypothyroidism

Licorice *(Glycyrrhiza glabra)*
Medicinal Parts: root
Uses: anti-inflammatory, antiviral, balances hormones, balances blood sugar, ulcers, tonifies adrenal glands

Lomatium *(Lomatium dissectum)* desert parsley
Medicinal Parts: root
Uses: viral and bacterial infections

Marshmallow root *(Althea officinalis)* marshmallow
Medicinal Parts: leaves, flowers, root
Uses: any inflamed mucosal tissue such as sore throat, ulcer

Milk thistle *(Carduus marianus)* holy thistle
Medicinal Parts: seeds
Uses: fatty liver, hepatitis, detoxification, poor fat digestion

Mullein *(Verbascum thapsus)* great mullein
Medicinal Parts: leaves for respiratory, flowers for oil infusions for ear complaints
Uses: irritated respiratory passageways, ear infection, cough, asthma, bronchitis

Myrrh *(Commiphora myrrha)* gum myrrh tree
Medicinal Parts: resin
Uses: antiseptic, cough, sores in mouth

Oatstraw *(Avena sativa)* oats
Medicinal Parts: grain, straw
Uses: nerve tonic, anxiety, stress, withdrawal from drug addictions

Onion *(Allium cepa)*
Medicinal Parts: bulb
Uses: vermicide, stimulates digestion, lowers blood pressure, antiparasitic, atherosclerosis

Oregon grape *(Mahonia aquifolium)*
Medicinal Parts: root
Uses: infections, stimulates liver detoxification, chronic skin conditions

Passion flower *(Passiflora incarnata)* passion vine
Medicinal Parts: leaf, stem, root
Uses: insomnia, nervousness, anxiety

Peppermint *(Mentha peperita)*
Medicinal Parts: leaves
Uses: cramps, poor digestion, abdominal pain, nausea, insomnia

Phytolacca *(Phytolacca decandra)* pokeroot
Medicinal Parts: root
Uses: swollen glands, throat infection, infected tonsils

Pipsissewa *(Chimaphila umbellata)* prince's pine
Medicinal Parts: entire plant
Uses: bladder and kidney infections, enlarged prostate

Raspberry *(Rubus strigosus)* wild red raspberry
Medicinal Parts: leaves, fruit
Uses: diarrhea, menstrual cramps

Red clover *(Trifolium pratense)*
Medicinal Parts: leaf, stem
Uses: cancer, hormone imbalance, mucous congestion

Reishi mushroom *(Ganoderma lucidum)*
Medicinal Parts: mushroom extract
Uses: immune stimulant, cancer

Sarsaparilla *(Smilax officinalis)* smilax
Medicinal Parts: rhizome
Uses: hormonal imbalance, enlarged prostate, syphilis, skin conditions

Saw palmetto *(Serenoa repens)*
Medicinal Parts: berries
Uses: enlarged prostate, ovarian cysts, acne

Scutellaria *(Scutellaria lateriflora)* skullcap
Medicinal Parts: leaf
Uses: anxiety, insomnia, muscular pain, viral infections

Shiitake mushroom *(Lentinus edodes)*
Medicinal Parts: mushroom extract
Uses: stimulates immune system, antiviral, HIV, cancer

Siberian ginseng *(Eleutherococcus senticosus)* ginseng
Medicinal Parts: root
Uses: adaptogen for physical or mental stress, sports training, fatigue, radiation, low blood pressure

Slippery elm *(Ulmus fulva)*
Medicinal Parts: inner bark
Uses: soothes irritated tissue such as an ulcer or sore throat

Stinging nettle *(Urtica dioica)* nettle
Medicinal Parts: entire plant
Uses: anemia, hayfever, allergies

St. John's wort *(Hypericum perforatum)* hypericum
Medicinal Parts: leaf, flowering tops
Uses: anti-inflammatory, antidepressant, antiviral

Tea tree *(Melaleuca alternifolia)*
Medicinal Parts: leaves
Uses: use externally for fungal and bacterial skin infections

Thuja *(Thuja occidentalis)* tree of life
Medicinal Parts: branches, leaves, bark
Uses: use externally for warts, skin problems

Tumeric *(Curcuma longa)*
Medicinal Parts: rhizome
Uses: anti-inflammatory, antimicrobial, anti-carcinogenic, increases bile secretion

Valerian *(Valeriana officinalis)*
Medicinal Parts: root
Uses: nervousness, stress, insomnia, depression

Witch hazel *(Hammamelis virginiana)* hazel nut
Medicinal Parts: bark, leaves
Uses: external application for bleeding, hemorrhoids, vaginitis

Yam *(Dioscorea villosa)* wild yam
Medicinal Parts: root
Uses: hormone imbalance, stomach cramps

Yarrow *(Achillea millefolium)*
Medicinal Parts: parts growing above ground
Uses: stop bleeding, heavy menses, anti-inflammatory

Yellow dock *(Rumex crispis)* curled dock
Medicinal Parts: roots
Uses: skin eruptions, anemia

Yohimbe *(Pausinystalia yohimbe)*
Medicinal Parts: bark
Uses: low sex drive, impotency

APPENDIX D

Natural Physician Healthy Diet Guidelines

There is no such thing as the perfect diet. We are all unique in our food preferences, digestive capabilities, nutritive requirements and body metabolism. The saying "What is a dessert for one person may be a poison for another" holds true. However, here are some dietary guidelines that can be applied universally.

1. **Rotate different foods into your diet.** Variety is very important to ensure a full supply of different nutrients, vitamins and minerals. Most people eat an average of the same twenty-five foods all the time. This increases the likelihood of becoming sensitive or intolerant to these food(s). Focus your menu on unprocessed foods. This should include a variety of plant-based foods such as vegetables, fruits, legumes, whole grains, seeds and nuts. Protein foods such as fish, legumes, soy, chicken breast and turkey breast should be consumed regularly.

2. **Eat a diet that focuses on natural foods.** Whenever possible eat certified organic foods. Pesticides, hormones and antibiotic residue accumulate over time in the body's tissues. These toxins can lead to degenerative changes in the body and the development of serious illness.

3. **Drink a minimum of six eight-ounce glasses of purified water daily.** Adequate amounts of water are necessary for proper cell metabolism and detoxification.

4. **Reduce intake of saturated fats.** They contain harmful fatty acids that damage the body and lead to illnesses such as cancer and heart disease. Saturated fat is found in animal products such as red meat and dairy products. Eat plant-based foods because they contain beneficial unsaturated fats.

5. **Minimize intake of fried foods.** They contain saturated fat and are hard to digest properly. Use cold-pressed oils such as

extra-virgin olive oil or flaxseed oil. If you must fry, never allow the oil to smoke—use a medium heat and use extra-virgin olive oil or a heat resistant oil such as cold-pressed peanut or sesame oil. For baking at temperatures above 350°F use butter.

6. **Minimize intake of refined sugars.** They interfere with proper functioning of the immune system. This includes table sugar or any other sweetener. Use honey, pure maple syrup, or fruit and fruit juices as sugar replacements.

7. **Minimize intake of table salt.** Most processed foods are loaded with sodium (salt). This leads to an imbalance between potassium and sodium in the body which may cause high blood pressure and heart disease.

8. **Increase fiber intake.** Fiber promotes efficient bowel elimination, stabilizes blood sugar release after a meal and promotes growth of beneficial bacteria in the colon. Sources of fiber include vegetables, fruits, seeds, legumes and seed husks such as psyllium. Oat bran and green leafy vegetables are great sources of fiber.

9. **Avoid foods with artificial sweeteners, preservatives, dyes and flavor enhancers.** Avoid foods or products containing artificial sweeteners such as Aspartame and Nutrasweet. Also avoid products containing preservatives such as MSG which can cause unfavorable reactions such as headaches. Preservatives may be toxic to the nervous system and damage the immune system.

10. **Drink fresh fruit and vegetable juices daily**. They contain an abundance of enzymes, vitamins and minerals.

11. **Eat smaller meals in the evening.** Digestive secretions and enzyme levels tend to decrease towards the end of the day. To ensure proper digestion eat larger meals for breakfast and lunch. In the evening eat smaller meals and foods that are easy to digest such as soups, and steamed and cooked vegetables.

12. **Eat in a calm atmosphere.** Take time to chew food thoroughly and relax after a meal. Listening to classical or other calming music helps to relax the body and promote efficient digestion.

13. **Treat yourself to a "goody" occasionally.** Moderation is the key. It is your general dietary habits that matter. Overzealous eating habits can create stress for the mind and body.

Natural Physician Meal Planner

Breakfast
Sample 1
Oatmeal or wholegrain cereal with rice milk or soy milk, sweetened with fresh fruit or honey, fresh almonds
Water, herbal tea or fresh fruit or vegetable juice

Sample 2
Poached eggs with wholegrain toast
Water, herbal tea or fresh fruit or vegetable juice

Lunch
Sample 1
Serving of fish (salmon, halibut, cod, shark or tuna), turkey, lamb or chicken breast; brown or white rice; quinoa or amaranth pasta; and a green leafy salad
Water, herbal tea or fresh fruit or vegetable juice

Sample 2
Cooked squash, eggplant, yams or baked tofu with wholegrain bread, beans and a green leafy salad
Water, herbal tea or fresh fruit or vegetable juice

Dinner
Sample 1
Soup or baked poultry or steamed fish, steamed or cooked vegetables, dinner rolls

Water, herbal tea or fresh fruit or vegetable juice
Sample 2
Light pasta dish, steamed or stir-fried vegetables
Water, herbal tea or fresh fruit or vegetable juice

Salads
An example of a nutritious salad includes combinations of romaine, red and green leaf lettuce, carrots, mushrooms, tomatoes, hearts of palm, cabbage, red onions, couscous, walnuts or sunflower seeds, radish, with an extra-virgin olive oil and vinegar dressing.

Snacks
• vegetable slices (e.g., carrots, cucumbers, cauliflower)
• fruits (e.g., watermelon, pears, plums, peaches, apricots, mango, blueberries)
• nuts and seeds (e.g., almonds, pecans, sunflower seeds)
• popcorn
• fresh fruit and vegetable juices
• rice cakes with nut butter toppings

Natural Physician Shake
Blend the following together:
3 cups of rice milk or soy milk
1 scoop of protein powder (preferably soy or spirulina base)
1 cup of fruit (e.g., strawberries, blueberries, raspberries)
1 tablespoon of flaxseed oil

APPENDIX E

Food Allergies and Sensitivities Elimination and Reintroduction Diet

The Elimination and Reintroduction diet is used to help identify food allergies and sensitivities. Symptoms of food allergies and sensitivities can vary depending on individual susceptibility. Common symptoms include but are not limited to the following:

- **Immune:** frequent colds and infections, autoimmune conditions
- **Digestive:** irritable bowel syndrome, constipation, bloating, diarrhea, Crohn's disease, ulcerative colitis, gall-bladder disease, hemorrhoids, colic
- **Urinary:** chronic bladder and kidney infections, bed-wetting
- **Respiratory:** bronchitis, sinusitis, ear infections
- **Gynecological:** vaginitis, fibrocystic breast disease
- **Musculoskeletal:** rheumatoid arthritis, osteoarthritis, fibromyalgia
- **Neurological:** migraine headaches
- **Other:** depression, fatigue, weight gain, weight loss

The strategy behind this diet is to eliminate the most common food sensitivities for a period of time. One can then re-introduce the foods one at a time to notice any adverse reactions. Most of the foods that are common causes of sensitivities are eaten on a daily basis in our society. Lack of variation in our diets leads to the immune system becoming sensitive to the foods that are eaten constantly. By avoiding our food sensitivities and by rotating different foods into the diet we can desensitize the immune system to these foods.

Careful observation and adherence to the following program is necessary to achieve accurate results in identifying food allergies and sensitivities:

1. Eliminate the following foods (common causes of food allergies and sensitivities) entirely for three to four weeks.

- **Dairy products**—cow's milk, cheese, ice cream, yogurt, food products containing casein or whey
  Replacement—rice milk
- **Wheat and wheat products**—breads, pastas, baked products with wheat
  Replacement—rice, spelt, amaranth, quinoa, millet
- **Soy products**
  Replacement—meat, chicken, turkey, fish
- **Eggs**
  Replacement—meat, chicken, turkey, fish
- **Citrus fruit**—oranges, lemons, citrus products, tomatoes
  Replacement—other fruit
- **Refined sugars**—table sugar, glucose, dextrose, corn syrup, fructose, maltose
  Replacement—organic maple syrup, honey, fruit and fruit juices
- **Food preservatives**—artificial flavors, sweeteners, sulfites, MSG
- **Alcohol and caffeine products**
  Replacement—herbal teas, grain beverages, fruit and vegetable juices, non-alcoholic beverages

2. After a period of three weeks reintroduce a category of the eliminated foods. Consume repeated servings of that food throughout the day. If there is a noticeable reaction to the food such as a headache or digestive reaction, discontinue the food at once. Record any reactions and stop eating any foods you react to. Every three days pick a different category of eliminated food and reintroduce it. *Only eat one category of food at any time, even if you do not react to it, until all eliminated foods have been tested.*

Note: Milk should be tested separately from cheese. All citrus fruits should be tried individually.

3. Avoid the foods that caused a reaction. Over the following months they can be reintroduced to see if the reaction has decreased or is gone.

Keep in mind that food sensitivities are a symptom of a damaged immune and digestive system. They can be neutralized by improving digestive function (see *Food Allergies and Sensitivities* section at the front of this book) and by herbal, homeopathic or Chinese medical treatment by a qualified practitioner.

Note: foods that cause known allergic reactions such as hives, swellings or constriction of the airway should not be consumed without the supervision of a physician.

APPENDIX F

Natural Physician Vitamin and Mineral Guide

Vitamins are organic substances that are essential for life: they are required for normal growth, metabolism and development. Vitamins act synergistically with enzymes and minerals to carry out normal metabolic processes. We must obtain most vitamins from plant, animal or nutritional supplements. Exceptions to this are vitamin A (converted from beta-carotene), vitamin D (converted from ultraviolet light by the skin), vitamin K (synthesized by intestinal bacteria) and a few B vitamins (synthesized by intestinal bacteria).

There are two main categories of vitamins: fat soluble and water soluble. Fat soluble vitamins (vitamins A, D, E and K) require fat particles for proper assimilation. They are stored in certain organs such as the liver for long periods of time (weeks to months). Water soluble vitamins (vitamin C and the B vitamins) do not need fat or food particles for absorption. They are absorbed quickly and excreted out of the body in the urine every two to three hours.

Minerals are organic substances that are also essential to life. Minerals are necessary to activate both vitamins and enzyme reactions. Since the body cannot manufacture minerals they must be consumed through the diet or by supplementation. Common minerals are calcium, magnesium, phosphorus, sodium and potassium. Also required, but only in minute amounts are trace minerals—such as manganese, selenium, boron, chromium, vanadium, silicon, copper, zinc, germanium, iodine, iron and molybdenum.

Vitamins and minerals should be used to supplement an existing healthy diet (refer to *Appendix D*) and if the diet is unhealthy it is even more critical to take supplements. One may ask why it is necessary to use supplements if a healthy diet is being followed. This is a question I have researched and I have come up with these conclusions:

- Most people in our society do not get optimal levels of nutrients from their diet. Supplementation is necessary to prevent nutrient deficiencies and promote optimal health.
- Modern agricultural techniques deplete much of the nutrient content of foods. Studies show that vegetables grown with chemical fertilizers and pesticides generally have fewer vitamins and minerals than organically grown vegetables.
- Much of the food we consume has been processed and therefore has reduced nutrient content.
- Fast food has become a way of life. The nutrition in these foods is much poorer in quality than whole foods.
- Pollution in the environment and foods increases the need for a higher nutritional status. Certain vitamins and minerals are needed to help detoxify cells and protect them from pollutants.
- Pharmaceutical medications are commonly used and many of these drugs are known to deplete the body of certain nutrients.
- Living in an age of high stress increases the requirement of certain vitamins and minerals.

Natural and Synthetic Vitamins

Natural vitamins are extracted from food sources. Synthetic vitamins are isolated chemicals that are manufactured in laboratories. The difference is that natural vitamins often contain a complex of additional compounds that work together to enhance the effectiveness of the single vitamin. For example, natural vitamin E contains the chemical d'alpha tocopherol but, unlike synthetic vitamin E, it also contains a group of other tocopherols that have many health benefits. Scientists have not yet identified all the health benefiting effects of natural vitamin-like compounds.

Dosages

The vitamin and mineral dosages given here are safe for those aged of sixteen years and older. Specific children's dosages are given when necessary. If dosages are not listed consult with a health care professional. *Note: U.S. RDAs (Recommended Daily Allowances) have been given.*

RDA

The Recommended Daily Allowance (RDA) levels were established in 1943 by the American National Council of Research. These recommendations were set as a standard for the daily amounts of vitamins and minerals required by a healthy person to prevent specific deficiency diseases (e.g., rickets, scurvy).

Nutritionally-oriented physicians are critical of RDA levels as they do not promote optimal health or take into account the special needs of individuals. For example, if you consume processed foods and are exposed to environmental pollution you have an increased need for many vitamins and minerals. The RDAs have been revised numerous times over the years and should be much higher in accordance with current nutritional research.

How to Use Vitamin and Mineral Supplements

Based on the diet of the average North American resident, pollution exposure, refined foods and stress levels, I recommend everyone take a daily multi-vitamin formula. Everyone has unique nutritional requirements, and certain individuals may require higher levels of specific nutrients than others. Those with acute or chronic illness will require higher levels of specific nutrients unique to their conditions (e.g., asthmatics require higher levels of magnesium, vitamin B6 and vitamin C). As well, those with disease promoting habits such as smoking require additional supplementation (e.g., all the antioxidants).

When following a vitamin-mineral program described in this book try to find formulas that contain the listed ingredients as it is more cost effective. I advise taking all supplements with meals for two reasons: it optimizes absorption and it is easier to make a routine of taking your supplements with meals. If you are taking more than one type of vitamin-mineral formula then spread out their use over the day instead of taking them all at once.

Remember, you do not have to have an illness to take vitamins and minerals. It is an excellent investment in your health to prevent nutritional deficiencies with quality vitamins and minerals.

I also recommend using a top quality concentrated plant food such as Enriching Green Factors by Natural Factors. The whole plant remains intact and provides many beneficial phyto chemicals. This type of product should be taken on a daily basis as part of a preventative supplementation program.

Natural Physician Multi-vitamin and Mineral Formula
Note: this is a recommended dosage range for adults.

Vitamins	Dosage
Beta-carotene	5,000–25,000 IU
Biotin	30–300 mcg
Choline	10–400 mg
Folic acid	400 mcg–1 mg
Inositol	10–100 mg
Niacin	10–100 mg
Niacinamide	10–30 mg
Pantothenic acid	25–300 mg
Vitamin A (retinol)	5,000–25,000 IU
(*do not exceed 4,000 IU daily if pregnant*)	
Vitamin B1 (thiamin)	10–100 mg
Vitamin B2 (riboflavin)	10–100 mg
Vitamin B6 (pyridoxine)	25–150 mg
Vitamin B12	400–800 mcg
Vitamin C (ascorbic acid)	100–1,000 mg
Vitamin D	100–400 IU
Vitamin E (d'alpha tocopherol)	200–400 IU
Vitamin K	60–300 mcg

Minerals	Dosage
Boron	0–3 mcg
Calcium	250–1000 mg
Chromium	150–200 mcg
Copper	0–3 mg
Iodine	0–150 mcg
Iron	0 mg
(*unless iron deficiency anemia or pregnant*)	
Magnesium	150–500 mg
Manganese	10–25 mg
Molybdenum	10–25 mcg

Minerals (continued)	Dosage
Potassium	150–500 mg
Selenium	100–200 mcg
Silica	25–200 mcg
Vanadium	50–100 mcg
Zinc	10–30 mg

Note: mg = milligrams   mcg = micrograms

Fat Soluble Vitamins

These vitamins should be taken with meals.

Vitamin A *(Retinol)*

About: Vitamin A occurs in two forms: retinol (from animal foods) and carotene (from plant and animal foods). It is most commonly measured in IU (International Units) or RE (Retinol Equivalents). Beta-carotene is converted by the body into vitamin A.

RDA: Females: 4,000 IU (800 RE) daily; Males: 5,000 IU (1,000 RE) daily

Sources: vegetables: carrots, yams, kale, collard greens, red pepper, sweet potatoes, parsley, spinach, mustard greens, broccoli, romaine lettuce, dark green and yellow vegetables; fruit: mangoes, cantaloupe, aprictos, papaya, peach, apples, avocado; animal products: liver, egg yolk, dairy products, white fish, cod liver oil

General Functions: general vision, night vision, body growth, skin health, immune system, reproduction, antioxidant

Indications: acne, wrinkles, boils, emphysema, hypothyroidism, eye disorders, respiratory tract infections, infections, menorrhagia, cervical dysplasia, wound healing, immune system enhancement, measles, ulcers

Deficiency: night blindness, growth impairment

Toxicity: bone pain, dry skin, enlarged spleen or liver, hair loss, gastro-intestinal upset, headache. Pregnant women or women planning conception should not take more than 4,000 IU daily. Those with liver disease should not supplement extra vitamin A. Additional vitamin A supplementation should be under the supervision of a physician.

Absorption: fat soluble—best taken with meals: acetate or palmitate are common forms
Therapeutic Dosage: 10,000 to 50,000 IU daily. High doses can be used on a short term basis for acute infections. Long-term use must be under the supervision of a physician.

Vitamin D (Cholecalciferol, Ergocalciferol)

About: There are two main food sources of vitamin D. Vitamin D2 (ergocalciferol) from plant sources and mainly used in nutritional supplements and vitamin D3 (cholecalciferol) from animal sources.
RDA: Adults: 200 IU daily; Infants/Children/Teenagers: 400 IU daily
Sources: sunlight, animal products: cod liver oil, mackerel, herring, salmon, tuna, vitamin-D-fortified milk, margarine, eggs, dark green leafy vegetables
General Functions: calcium and phosphorus absorption and metabolism
Indications: formation of bone and teeth, absorption and utilization of calcium, preventing osteoporosis, preventing breast cancer, psoriasis, colon cancer
Deficiency: rickets in children—stunted growth and malformation of bone structure; osteomalacia in adults—softening of bone leading to increased bone fractures; osteoporosis
Toxicity: kidney damage, calcium deposits
Absorption: fat soluble—best taken with meals
Therapeutic Dosage: 200 to 800 IU daily. People not exposed to sunlight need a minimum of 400 IU daily.

Vitamin E (Tocopherol)

About: Composed of eight different substances called tocopherols. Known for its antioxidant activity.
RDA: 15 IU
Sources: wheat germ, vegetable oils, whole wheat, green leafy vegetables, nuts, eggs, Brussels sprouts, soybeans, beans
General Functions: protects cells from damage (antioxidant), protects red blood cells, important for reproductive functions
Indications: blood clots, scar dissolving, burns, leg cramps, heart disease, fibrocystic breast disease, menopausal hot flashes, cataracts, vaginal dryness, lupus, cancer, diabetes, macular degen-

eration, multiple sclerosis, arthritis, wound healing, heart disease
Deficiency: altered reflexes, decreased red blood cell life, reproductive disorders, decreased skin sensation
Toxicity: digestive upset
Absorption: fat soluble—best taken with meals
Therapeutic Dosage: 400 to 1,200 IU

Vitamin K *(Phylloquinone)*

About: Known for its role in blood clotting.
RDA: Females: 65 mcg; Males: 85 mcg
Sources: green leafy vegetables, soy lecithin, liver, Brussels sprouts, asparagus, alfalfa, safflower oil, kelp, egg yolk, cauliflower, soybeans, broccoli, kale, cabbage, asparagus, lettuce, spinach, green tea, synthesized by intestinal bacteria
General Functions: blood clotting, bone formation
Indications: celiac disease, colitis, osteoporosis, nausea
Deficiency: prolonged bleeding, bruising
Toxicity: high bilirubin levels, anemia, itchy skin
Absorption: fat soluble—best taken with meals
Therapeutic Dosage: may be supplemented at 100 to 500 mcg

Water Soluble Vitamins

Vitamin B1 *(Thiamine)*

About: Known for its effects on the nervous system and energy pathways. It needs to be replaced daily.
RDA: 1.5 mg daily
Sources: brewer's yeast, soybeans, nuts and seeds, wholegrain cereals, wheat, brown rice, oats, liver, organic meats, egg yolk, synthesized by intestinal bacteria
General Functions: metabolism of carbohydrates into energy and nerve function
Indications: depression, airsickness or seasickness, herpes zoster, alcoholism, neurological conditions such as Bell's palsy, sciatica, trigeminal neuralgia
Deficiency: fatigue, loss of appetite, depression, nerve and heart degeneration, irritability

Toxicity: none really known
Absorption: water soluble—best taken with other B vitamins with or without food
Therapeutic Dosage: 10 to 100 mg daily

Vitamin B2 *(Riboflavin)*

About: Necessary for growth and energy production.
RDA: 1.7 mg daily
Sources: dairy products, organ meats, eggs, brewer's and torula yeast, soybeans, spinach, whole grains, green leafy vegetables
General Functions: metabolism of carbohydrates into energy, normal growth
Indications: fatigue, vision, headache, muscle cramps, cataracts, macular degeneration, alcoholism, sore mouth, lips or tongue
Deficiency: cracks in corners of mouth, red and burning eyes, swollen tongue, poor vision
Toxicity: none really known
Absorption: water soluble—best taken with other B vitamins with or without food
Therapeutic Dosage: 10 to 100 mg daily

Vitamin B3 *(Niacin)*

About: The body can manufacture its own from the amino acid tryptophan with the help of vitamins B1, B2 and B6. It is important for development of sex hormones and energy.
RDA: 15 to 20 mg daily
Sources: wheat, liver, milk, legumes, eggs, broccoli, avocados, figs, prunes, torula yeast, brewer's yeast, peanuts, chicken, turkey, beef, fish, synthesized by intestinal bacteria
General Functions: metabolism of carbohydrates into energy; synthesis of fatty acids and steroid hormone production; detoxification; lowers blood triglycerides and cholesterol levels; helps with absorption of chromium
Indications: digestive problems, skin conditions, migraine headaches, high blood pressure, diarrhea, Ménière's syndrome, fatigue, canker sores, bad breath, high cholesterol and triglycerides, osteoarthritis, depression, diabetes, mental illness

Deficiency: skin inflammation, dementia, diarrhea, memory loss, headaches, weakness

Toxicity: non-toxic below 100 mg; flushing of the skin called niacin flush can occur with niacin (not with niacinamide or inositol hexaniacinate form)—it is not serious and usually disappears in thirty minutes. Doses above 100 mg may result in increased blood sugar, increased uric acid levels, liver toxicity and prolonged bleeding.

Absorption: water soluble—best taken with meals (to reduce chances of a flushing reaction) and other B vitamins

Therapeutic Dosage: 300 to 2,000 mg daily

Vitamin B5 *(Pantothenic Acid)*

About: Important for cell growth and the adrenal (stress) glands.

RDA: none has been given but 4 to 7 mg is estimated

Sources: eggs, liver, turkey, soy, salmon, brewer's yeast, chicken, green vegetables, synthesized by intestinal bacteria

General Functions: energy, hormone and blood production

Indications: infections, fatigue, adverse effects of antibiotics and postoperative shock, allergies, adrenal gland function, high cholesterol and triglycerides, rheumatoid arthritis, allergies

Deficiency: low blood pressure, hair loss, burning foot pain, fatigue

Toxicity: none known

Absorption: water soluble—best taken with other B vitamins with or without food

Therapeutic Dosage: 100 to 2,000 mg daily

Vitamin B6 *(Pyridoxine)*

About: Higher requirement with high protein diets. Needed for proper B12 absorption and production of stomach acid. Known for its effects on energy pathways, nerve function and detoxification pathways.

RDA: 1.6 to 2 mg daily

Sources: grains, egg yolk, brewer's yeast, canteloupe, cabbage, oats, peas, peanuts, walnuts, brown rice, bananas, nuts, seeds, potatoes, organ meats, soybeans, fish, synthesized by intestinal bacteria

General Functions: protein, carbohydrate and fat metabolism; normal growth; steroid hormone metabolism, red blood cell formation

Indications: skin disorders, nausea, muscle spasms, carpal tunnel syndrome, PMS, ADHD, asthma, osteoporosis, kidney stones, atherosclerosis, depression, diabetes, epilepsy

Deficiency: anemia, nerve disorders, fluid retention, tongue inflammation and scalp flaking

Toxicity: dosages over 200 mg daily have been reported to cause sensory nerve damage

Absorption: water soluble—best taken with other B vitamins with or without meals. Riboflavin (B2) and magnesium are needed for proper utilization of B6.

Therapeutic Dosage: 50 to 250 mg daily.

Vitamin B12 *(Cobalamin)*

About: A major vitamin for the nervous system and red blood cell formation. Often deficient in the elderly and strict vegetarians.

RDA: 2 mcg

Sources: organ meats, beef, pork, sardines, eggs, dairy products

General Functions: proper cell replication, development of red blood cells, nerve function, synergistic action with folic acid

Indications: anemia, fatigue, nervous system disorders, poor concentration and memory, deltoid bursitis, asthma, shingles, sciatica, AIDS, Alzheimer's, depression, diabetic neuropathy, multiple sclerosis

Deficiency: fatigue, poor memory, numbness, anemia, swollen tongue, spinal degeneration, depression

Toxicity: no real toxicity except possibly acne as a side-effect

Absorption: water soluble—sublingual or injection are preferred for severe deficiencies. Best when used with folic acid.

Therapeutic Dosage: 100 to 2,000 mcg daily

Biotin

About: Involved with metabolism of carbohydrates, fat and protein.

RDA: There is no RDA but 30 to 300 mcg is recommended

Sources: organ meats, egg yolk, nuts, milk, unpolished rice, kidney, beans, soybeans, legumes, cheese, synthesized by intestinal bacteria

General Functions: carbohydrate and fat metabolism, amino acid metabolism, cell replication

Indications: prevents non-genetic baldness, muscle pain, eczema, dermatitis, cradle cap, diabetes, poor nail growth

Deficiency: hair loss, depression, loss of appetite, loss of memory, inflamed tongue, dry skin, skin rash

Toxicity: none known

Absorption: water soluble

Therapeutic Dosage: 300 to 3,000 mcg daily

Choline

About: This is a lipotropic agent like inositol that works to metabolize fat and cholesterol and manufacture the neurotransmitter acetylcholine.

RDA: none given but estimated at 500 mg daily

Sources: green leafy vegetables, yeast, egg yolks, wheat germ, heart, soybeans, legumes, cauliflower

General Functions: fat and cholesterol metabolism; brain cell health; nervous system health

Indications: memory loss, high cholesterol, fatty liver, Alzheimer's, bipolar depression

Deficiency: cirrhosis and fatty deposits on liver, possible memory loss

Toxicity: none known

Absorption: water soluble—best when taken with other B vitamins, specially inositol. Can be taken as part of phosphatidylcholine supplement.

Therapeutic Dosage: 500 to 1,000 mg daily or as phosphatidylcholine at a dosage of 5,000 to 10,000 mg

Folic Acid

About: Required for proper development of the nervous system, cell division and red blood cell formation.

RDA: Females: 200 mcg daily; Males: 180 mcg daily

Sources: green leafy vegetables, carrots, liver, canteloupe, apricots, pumpkin, avocado, whole wheat, rye, fruit, organ meat, soybeans, oats and rice, kale, spinach, broccoli, brewer's yeast
General Functions: proper cell replication, development of red blood cells, nerve function, synergistic action with vitamin B12
Indications: breast milk production, food poisoning, skin rashes, prevents birth defects, prevents canker sores, anemia, prevents neural tube defects, cervical dysplasia, osteoporosis, cardiovascular disease, gout, gingivitis, depression, atherosclerosis, AIDS, fatigue, Parkinson's disease, restless leg syndrome, inflammatory bowel disease
Deficiency: anemia, memory impairment, infertility, neural tube defects
Toxicity: none known
Absorption: water soluble—best when taken in combination with vitamin B12. Injections of folic acid are most effective.
Therapeutic Dosage: 800 mcg to 10 mg daily

Inositol

About: Metabolizes fat and cholesterol. Combines with choline to form lecithin.
RDA: none given but estimated at 1 gram daily
Sources: brewer's yeast, liver, canteloupe, grapefruit, raisins, wheat germ, peanuts, cabbage, lima beans
General Functions: fat and cholesterol metabolism; brain cell health; hair growth
Indications: high cholesterol, hair loss, eczema, nervousness, fatty liver, depression, diabetes
Deficiency: eczema
Toxicity: none known
Absorption: water soluble—best taken with other B vitamins. The inositol hexaniacinate form avoids possible flushing reaction.
Therapeutic Dosage: 500 to 3,000 mg daily

PABA *(Para-aminobenzoic acid)*

About: Considered a new member of the B family.
RDA: none given

Sources: brewer's yeast, liver, whole grains, rice, bran, wheat germ, molasses
General Functions: involved in formation of folic acid
Indications: skin health, sunburns (there is a debate as to whether it's a safe sunscreen), natural hair color restoration, scleroderma, vitiligo
Deficiency: eczema, depression, irritability
Toxicity: possibly nausea or vomiting
Absorption: water soluble—best taken with other B vitamins with or without meals
Therapeutic Dosage: 30 to 1,000 mg daily

Vitamin C

About: Animals synthesize their own vitamin C but humans need an external source. It is essential for wound healing and immune function.
RDA: 60 mg daily; 100 mg daily for smokers
Sources: citrus fruits, peaches, melons, rose-hips, green peppers, tomatoes, potatoes, guava, green leafy vegetables, broccoli, Brussels sprouts
General Function: connective tissue formation, bone health, wound healing, aids in allergic responses, steroid hormone production, immune function, antioxidant, enhances iron absorption
Indications: wound healing, burns, bleeding gums, high cholesterol, infections, cancer protection, colds, allergies, diabetes, gout, spinal disk degeneration, infertility, glaucoma, asthma, candidiasis, cataracts, cervical dysplasia, hepatitis, hypertension, infertility, macular degeneration, arthritis
Deficiency: poor wound healing, hemorrhage, loose teeth, friable blood vessels, gum swelling and bleeding, skin thickening, bruising
Toxicity: high doses (varies for each individual) can cause diarrhea
Absorption: water soluble—take any time. Natural source is better absorbed than chemical source. It is more efficient when taken with high amounts of bioflavonoids.
Therapeutic Dosage: 1,000 mg to highest dosage tolerated

Minerals

Boron

About: Known for its effect on estrogen and bone mass.

RDA: none yet

Sources: honey, non-citrus fruits (apples, grapes, peaches, cherries), green leafy vegetables, nuts, legumes

General Function: production of steroid hormones which may help with bone mass

Indications: osteoporosis, menopause, arthritis

Deficiency: postmenopausal bone loss

Toxicity: unknown

Absorption: best taken with meals

Therapeutic Dosage: 1 to 5 mg daily

Calcium

About: Most abundant mineral in the body. Known for its role in bone formation, muscle contraction and neurotransmitter function.

RDA: Females and pregnant females: 1200 mg daily, Males: 800 mg daily

Sources: dairy products, sesame seeds, almonds and other nuts, sardines, trout, kelp, broccoli, parsley, collard greens, dried beans, kale, spinach, tofu

General Function: bone formation, muscle and nerve conduction, blood clotting and heart contraction, works synergistically with magnesium

Indications: osteoporosis, osteomalacia, rickets, muscle cramps and spasms, hypertension, pregnancy

Deficiency: osteoporosis (decreased bone density), osteomalacia (softening of bone), muscle cramps

Toxicity: possible kidney damage and digestive problems such as constipation

Absorption: best when taken with meals. Taken in conjunction with magnesium in a 2:1 or 1:1 ratio. Chelated calcium, calcium citrate and microcrystalline hydroxyapatite (MCHA) are most efficiently absorbed.

Therapeutic Dosage: 500 to 1,500 mg daily

Chromium

About: Useful for balancing blood sugar.

RDA: no RDA but the recommended dosage is 50 to 200 mcg daily

Sources: brewer's yeast, legumes, clams, chicken, corn oil, calf liver, mushrooms, whole grains

General Function: regulates blood sugar and promotes lean muscle mass, reduces craving for sweets

Indications: arteriosclerosis, diabetes, hypoglycemia, athletic training, weight loss, high cholesterol, acne, high triglycerides

Deficiency: weight gain, poor glucose tolerance, nerve inflammation, high cholesterol

Toxicity: none known

Absorption: chromium picolinate or polynicotinate, formula should contain a form of niacin to be most effective

Therapeutic Dosage: 200 to 600 mcg

Cobalt

About: Assimilated as part of vitamin B12.

RDA: about 1 mcg daily

Sources: organ meats, peanuts, peas, sardines, salmon

General Function: used to form vitamin B1

Indications: none

Deficiency: rare

Toxicity: possible thyroid growth, congestive heart failure and anemia

Absorption: best taken as part of vitamin B12 supplement with meals

Therapeutic Dosage: 3 to 10 mcg daily as part of B12 supplement

Copper

About: Known for its synergistic effect with zinc. Promotes connective tissue formation.

RDA: no RDA but an adequate dosage is 2 to 3 mg daily

Sources: sesame seeds, cashews, oysters, bran, pumpkin seeds, legumes, poultry, almonds, avocados, mushrooms, seafood

General Function: helps in enzyme systems, neurotransmitter production, connective tissue formation, detoxification

Indications: anemia, edema, skeletal defects, rheumatoid arthritis, osteoporosis

Deficiency: anemia, abnormal connective tissue, nervous system disorders, depigmentation, hair loss, lowered immune system function

Toxicity: liver damage and diarrhea in small children, depression, joint pain. Dosage above 10 mg may cause nausea and vomiting in children and adults.

Absorption: best taken with meals—should be taken in a 1:8 ratio with zinc

Therapeutic Dosage: 1 to 4 mg daily

Coenzyme Q10

About: Known for positive effects on energy production and cardiovascular health.

RDA: none known

Sources: beef heart, sardines, peanuts, spinach, mackerel, salmon

General Function: energy production, antioxidant, boost immune system function, connective tissue formation, heart function

Indications: congestive heart failure, mitral valve prolapse, angina, cardiomyopathy, ischemia, peridontal disease, hypertension, heart disease, gingivitis, cancer, fatigue, metastic breast cancer, diabetes, athletic performance

Deficiency: coronary heart disease

Toxicity: none known

Absorption: capsule or sublingual

Therapeutic Dosage: 30 to 300 mg daily

Fluoride

About: Known for its prevention of dental disease. Controversy over whether supplementation in any form is necessary or not.

RDA: none but estimated to be about 1.5 to 4 mg daily

Sources: seafood, black tea, toothpaste, water

General Function: connective tissue formation and calcium deposits
Indications: dental cavities
Deficiency: possibly teeth decay
Toxicity: digestive upset, arthritic-like symptoms, mottling of teeth, possible lowered immune function
Absorption: best taken with meals
Therapeutic Dosage: 1 to 5 mg daily

Germanium

About: Known for immune stimulation and energy production.
RDA: unknown
Sources: ginseng, water chestnut, pearl barley, garlic, sushi, chlorella, barley, garlic, comfrey, aloe, tuna, beans, shiitake mushroom, onion
General Function: energy production
Indications: cancer, fatigue, AIDS
Deficiency: unknown
Toxicity: unknown
Absorption: best taken with meals
Therapeutic Dosage: about 1.5 mg daily

Iodine

About: Known for its necessity in thyroid function.
RDA: 100 to 150 mcg daily
Sources: table salt, fish, kelp, onions, dairy products, iodized table salt, seafood—especially seaweed
General Function: production of thyroid hormones
Indications: goiter, hypothyroidism, fibrocystic breast syndrome
Deficiency: low thyroid function, goiter, cretinism, growth retardation, newborn hypothyroidism
Toxicity: skin rash, depression, worsening of acne, hyperthyroid
Absorption: raw cauliflower, kale, Brussels sprouts, spinach and turnips may interfere with iodine utilization by the thyroid gland. Cooking these foods deactivates this effect.
Therapeutic Dosage: 0.5 to 1 mg daily

Iron

About: Important for the production of red blood cells to carry oxygen.

RDA: Females: 15 mg daily; Males: 10 mg daily

Sources: many sources including organ meats, beef, seafood, egg yolk, beans, dark green leafy vegetables, peaches, pears, blackstrap molasses, wheat bran, parsley, sunflower seeds

General Function: formation of red blood cells to carry oxygen

Deficiency: anemia, fatigue, sore tongue, skin problems, decreased growth, lowered immune system function, heart problems, hair loss, restless leg syndrome, menorrhagia

Indications: iron deficiency anemia

Toxicity: called hemochromatosis where excess iron levels cause liver and pancreatic damage, loss of menses, sterility, joint pain, heart damage, cancer and lowered immunity. Children are prone to iron toxicity which can cause vomiting, shock, intestinal damage and liver failure

Absorption: best when taken with meals. Iron aspartate, gluconate and fumerate are good sources. Avoid iron sulfate as it can cause constipation. Take with vitamin C to enhance absorption.

Therapeutic Dosage: 10 to 50 mg daily. Iron should only be supplemented if iron deficiency has been diagnosed by a blood test. Otherwise, supplementation can lead to toxic levels which may cause cardiovascular or liver disease.

Magnesium

About: Known for its benefit for muscle, heart and nerve contraction.

RDA: Females: 300 mg daily; Males: 350 mg daily

Sources: nuts (almonds, cashews, brazil nuts), wheat germ, bran, buckwheat, corn, peas, figs, bananas, green leafy vegetables, carrots, tofu, legumes

General Function: bone formation, nerve and muscle transmission, energy production, activates B vitamins, protein synthesis, works synergistically with calcium

Indications: heart disease, muscle cramps, neurological disorders, fatigue, hypertension, asthma, osteoporosis, diabetes,

migraine headache, fibromyalgia, kidney stones, pre-eclampsia of pregnancy, PMS, mitral valve prolapse, hypoglycemia
Deficiency: muscle weakness and cramping, high blood pressure
Toxicity: kidney damage, diarrhea, heart arrhythmia
Absorption: best when taken with meals. Should be taken with calcium. Magnesium aspartate, a chelated form with amino acid absorbs well. Magnesium glycinate does not cause diarrhea.
Therapeutic Dosage: 500 to 1,500 mg daily

Manganese
About: Used to activate enzyme systems in the body.
RDA: no RDA but an adequate daily intake would be 5 mg daily
Sources: whole grains, nuts, blueberries, blackberries, tea, green leafy vegetables, peas, beets, avocados, whole grains, seaweeds
General Function: formation of bone, cartilage and connective tissue; antioxidant; formation of neurotransmitters
Indications: dizziness, fatigue, osteoporosis, poor memory, sprains, strains, epilepsy, diabetes
Deficiency: uncommon
Toxicity: nervous system disorders
Absorption: manganese carbonate, manganese oxide, manganese chloride are good sources. High calcium or phosphorus intake can hinder absorption.
Therapeutic Dosage: 5 to 40 mg daily

Molybdenum
About: Important for fat and carbohydrate metabolism.
RDA: no RDA but typically 150 to 500 mcg daily
Sources: lamb, green beans, lentils, squash, strawberries, carrots, dark green leafy vegetables
General Function: detoxification
Indications: anemia, asthma due to sulfite allergy, cancer prevention, Wilson's disease
Deficiency: may interfere with normal body development
Toxicity: unknown, high amounts may interfere with copper utilization or cause gout

Absorption: best taken with meals
Therapeutic Dosage: 200 to 500 mcg daily

Phosphorus
About: Bone formation.
RDA: 600 to 800 mg daily
Sources: egg yolk, cheese, milk, chicken, beef, whole grains, legumes, nuts, asparagus, salmon
General Function: energy production, formation of bones and teeth
Indications: rare
Deficiency: —muscle weakness, irritability, digestive problems
Toxicity: possible kidney damage
Absorption: take with or without meals
Therapeutic Dosage: 600 to 1,000 mg daily

Potassium
About: Important for nerve and heart regulation.
RDA: 1.8 to 5 g daily
Sources: fruits and vegetables, apples, oranges, carrots, fish, whole grains, legumes, meat, poultry
General Function: electrical activity, heart function, acid-base balance, kidney and adrenal function
Indications: high blood pressure, heart arrhythmia
Deficiency: abnormal skin sensations, heartbeat irregularities, muscle weakness
Toxicity: nausea, vomiting, diarrhea. Those with kidney disorders or on potassium sparing diuretics for hypertension should only supplement potassium under a physician's supervision.
Absorption: take with or without meals
Therapeutic Dosage: 1.8 to 5 g daily

Selenium
About: A powerful antioxidant.
RDA: 70 mcg
Sources: organ meats, fish, whole grains, brewer's yeast, kidney, liver, tomatoes, broccoli
General Function: antioxidant, chelates heavy metals, thyroid

hormone production

Indications: fatigue, cancer prevention, cardiovascular disease, macular degeneration, viral infections, arthritis

Deficiency: heart disease, breakdown of cartilage and muscle, thyroid failure

Toxicity: hair loss, nail loss, white spots on nails, nausea, vomiting, hyper reflexes, muscle weakness, skin rash

Absorption: best taken with meals

Therapeutic Dosage: 200 to 500 mcg daily

Silicon

About: Involved with formation of connective tissue such as the skin, bones, ligaments and tendons.

RDA: no RDA but 5 to 30 mg is an adequate daily intake

Sources: rice, bran, grains, leafy vegetables, horsetail, oatmeal

General Function: production of connective tissue, bones and teeth

Indications: brittle nails, osteoporosis, brittle hair

Deficiency: inadequate bone development

Toxicity: unknown

Absorption: best taken with meals

Therapeutic Dosage: 1 to 2 mg daily

Sodium

About: Important for nerve impulse and water regulation in the tissue.

RDA: 1.1 to 3.3 g daily

Sources: table salt, processed foods, seafood, chicken, beef, milk, many vegetables

General Function: electrical activity, blood pressure, acid/base balance

Indications: dehydration

Deficiency: rare

Toxicity: high blood pressure, subarachanoid hemorrhage, vomiting, diarrhea, kidney damage

Absorption: take with or without meals

Therapeutic Dosage: used therapeutically in emergency situations only

Vanadium
About: Aids in blood sugar balancing.
RDA: unknown but 10 to 60 mcg is an adequate daily intake
Sources: fish, mushrooms, parsley, dill, black pepper
General Function: blood sugar regulation
Indications: diabetes
Deficiency: possible impaired growth
Toxicity: possible kidney damage, possible manic depression at very high dosages
Absorption: best taken with meals
Therapeutic Dosage: 50 to 100 mcg daily

Zinc
About: Involved in the immune system and reproductive organs.
RDA: 15 mg daily
Sources: dairy products, shellfish, meat, seafood (oysters, fish), pumpkin seeds, eggs, green leafy vegetables, wheat bran, fruit
General Function: works synergistically with vitamin A and copper, normal growth, antioxidant, stomach acid production, boosts immune system function
Indications: wound healing, loss of taste, infertility, enlarged prostate, mental disorders, acne, ulcer, arthritis, poor taste sensation, anorexia nervosa, alcoholism, arthritis, macular degeneration, Wilson's disease
Deficiency: skin rash, depression, poor wound healing, decreased sperm count, poor sense of smell and taste, diarrhea
Toxicity: impaired immune system function, anemia, nausea, skin rash, alcohol intolerance
Absorption: best taken with meals. Should be taken at a 8:1 ratio with copper. Zinc picolinate or aspartate are best absorbed.
Therapeutic Dosage: 20 to 100 mg daily. *Note: doses above 50 mg should not be taken on a long-term basis.*

Appendix G

Natural Physician Guide to Choosing Quality Supplements

As with any product, it is quality that counts. Knowing how to choose well from the increasing variety of supplements available can be confusing. Investing in your health should be a rewarding experience. The supplements you choose need to be the highest quality to ensure effectiveness.

Many of my patients have tried certain brands of supplements before coming to me. Often the type of supplement is known to be beneficial for their condition (e.g., milk thistle for elevated liver enzymes), but there was no improvement because they were taking supplements of poor quality or an incorrect dosage. After prescribing the same supplement but of higher quality we often find the desired health result(s).

Some people believe that natural supplements are not efficacious based on their personal experience. In a way they are right, as many of the supplements people use are of no medicinal value. Be cautious, the quality of supplements varies greatly between manufacturers. To safeguard against this problem you must educate yourself. This appendix will provide you with the guidelines I believe are important in choosing a quality supplement from a reputable company.

Quality of Supplements

There are a number of factors to consider to ensure the supplement you purchase is of optimum quality.

- The supplement label should clearly state the ingredients and amounts. For example, calcium citrate 500 mg per capsule. It should also state if any potential allergenic substances are contained in the product (e.g., red dye #4). If a product does not clearly state the ingredients and amounts do not purchase it.

• The supplement company should be able to provide documentation of product analysis on request. The analysis confirms the potency and purity of the supplement and protects the consumer from contaminants such as parasites, bacteria, pesticides and heavy metals. Look for manufacturers that use high-tech analytical processes such as the HPLC method.

• Herbal products should state the percent standardized extract of known active compounds in addition to the popular dosage in milligrams. For example, St. John's wort is standardized for a level of 0.3% hypericin and is commonly prescribed at 300 mg two to three times daily. Hypericin is a known active compound in St. John's wort. Many of the herbal products have known active compounds, although not all herbal medicines have known standardized extract values.

• Combination formulas can be useful as different vitamins and herbs can exert synergistic effects. However, many companies add unnecessary ingredients in these combination formulas which render them useless and a waste of money. To ensure the combination product you buy will be effective, look for educational material that accompanies the product to explain the action of each ingredient. As well, compare the formula to the information provided by reputable natural health care professionals as described in books.

Qualities of a Reputable Supplement Company

When choosing a company from which to purchase supplements, look at the following:

• years of experience in the industry
• educational material provided
• product origins provided: e.g., organic herbal farms
• analysis of products—all products should be routinely tested for purity and potency by modern scientific technology
• research—look for companies committed to research and scientific validation of natural health care products. These types of companies provide their consumer with current information on product development and usage. They also help advance the growing field of natural medicine.

Natural Factors

In my experience, Natural Factors is an excellent example as one of the world leaders in quality nutritional supplements. For more than thirty-five years they have harvested, prepared and distributed herbal remedies, vitamin and mineral supplements, and other natural health products throughout North America, Europe and Asia.

Natural Factors is known for its dedication to providing educational material for natural food stores and has health care professionals on staff to provide expert advice on product usage.

Unlike most companies, Natural Factors produces many of its own certified organic herbal products grown at Factor Farms in BC's Okanagan region and pollen at Factor Farms in the Peace River Valley.

Natural Factors has an independent state-of-the-art laboratory where all products are tested to ensure quality, potency and purity. As well, scientific research is a high priority, allowing manufacturers to provide consumers with higher quality products and advances the scientific understanding and validation of natural medicine.

Glossary

Absorption—the passage of nutrients from the digestive system into the bloodstream.

Acetyl-L-Carnitine—composed of an ester group attached to the vitamin carnitine. It is thought to serve as a precursor to the neurotransmitter acetylcholine for effective neuron function. It may help restore cell membrane stability. Currently being investigated for its effectiveness in Alzheimer's disease.

Acupuncture—a component of Chinese medicine that is based on the theory that the body has several main energy channels. Illness or disharmony arises when there is a blockage of energy (chi) flow in one or more of these channels. Fine needles are inserted into or applied to one or more of the more than 500 acupuncture point(s) on these channels to move the disrupted energy flow.

Adaptogen—a substance that helps the body increase its resistance to physical or mental stress.

Adrenal glands—a pair of glands located on top of the kidneys. Stress hormones such as epinephrine, cortisol, DHEA and others are produced by these glands.

Amaranth—an ancient grain with seeds similar in size to millet. It is high in protein and amaranth flour is gluten-free and is commonly used as a wheat alternative.

Amino acid—one of twenty individual building blocks of protein. Each amino acid when taken individually can produce different biochemical effects.

Anti-inflammatory—a substance that blocks or lessens inflammation.

Antioxidant—a substance that protects other cells from oxidation or free radical damage. Examples of well known antioxidants include vitamins A, C and E, beta-carotene and selenium.

Astringent—a substance that has a binding or constricting effect.

Atherosclerosis—the deposition and build-up of plaque and fatty substances onto artery walls. This leads to narrowing of the artery and decreased blood flow.

Autoimmune condition—a condition where the body's immune system reacts against its own tissues causing them damage.

Bach flower remedy—developed by medical doctor Edward Bach in the early 1900s, these are extracts of various flowers or buds of common plants that are prepared into a homeopathic dilution. These medicines have their main action on mental and emotional imbalances.

Betaine HCl—a supplemental source of stomach hydrochloric acid that aids in digestion.

Biofeedback—a technique used to help one gain control over their nervous system and bodily functions to re-establish health. Electronic machines are used to monitor metabolic changes (heart rate, muscle tension and temperature change), while consciously visualizing or relating the patient learns to correct internal imbalances.

Bioflavonoid—a vitamin-like supplement that exhibits effects similar to vitamin C. They are derived from the pigments of fruits and flowers such as orange and lemon peels. They are also known as vitamin P complex.

Blue-green algae—extracted blue-green algae contains amino acids, vitamins and minerals to repair damaged tissue. It also contains chlorophyll that acts to detoxify the body.

Bovine cartilage—an extract of bovine tracheal cartilage used in the treatment of cancer and arthritis.

Bromelain—an enzyme complex extracted from pineapple. When taken with food it helps to digest proteins. If taken between meals it has an anti-inflammatory effect.

Carbohydrates—sugar and starchy foods.

Cartilage—connective tissue in the joints that absorb shock.

Charcoal capsules—activated charcoal used to adsorb toxins. Can be used internally or externally.

Chelated minerals—a process where minerals are made into a more efficiently absorbed chelating agents such as EDTA.

Chelation therapy—the use of chelating agents in an intravenous form to bind heavy metals and other toxins and excrete them out of the body. It is now being used for conditions such as coronary artery disease where plaque build-up is a problem.

Chiropractic—a system of health enhancement based on the relationship between the spine and nervous system. Specific adjustments to the spine are used to ensure optimal nerve, circulatory and immune function.

Chlorophyll—a pigment that gives plants their green color. It has detoxifying and blood building qualities.

Cholesterol—a fat soluble substance required for proper cell functions. Excess cholesterol can be harmful.

Creatine—a nutrient that occurs naturally in the body. It is composed of three amino acids—arginine, glycine and methionine. Its use is popular among athletes for its ability to enhance performance and training recovery.

DHEA (Dehydroepiandosterone)—a hormone produced by the adrenal glands that is a precursor to many of the hormones in the body. Currently being studied for its benefit on aging, hormone deficiency illness and chronic illness such as lupus and arthritis.

DNA—abbreviation for deoxyribonucleic acid, a substance found in the cells and which contains the genetic code.

Diuretic—a substance that increases the excretion of urine.

Enzyme—a catalyst for biochemical reactions in the body. Used by the body in digestion.

Essential fatty acids—fatty acids required for normal bodily functioning and that the body cannot produce on its own. They are linoleic and linolenic acid.

Estrogen—a hormone responsible for female characteristics.

Fat soluble—able to dissolve in fats and oils. Vitamins A, D, K and E need fat to be properly absorbed.

Food allergy—a reaction to a food that involves an immune response. Resulting symptoms can include hives, anaphylaxis (closing of the windpipe), runny nose and stomach disturbances.

Food sensitivity—a reaction to a food that does not have a measurable immune system reaction. Common reactions can include rashes, digestive problems, headaches, mood changes, insomnia and many other symptoms.

Free radical—a highly reactive molecule due to an unpaired electron and which can cause cell and tissue damage. They are formed from heated oils and fats, environmental pollution and as a by-product of metabolic reactions within the body. They are neutralized by naturally occurring enzymes in the body and by antioxidants.

Glandular—concentrated protein extracts from the glands of bovine and pork sources. They are used to nourish the same type of gland that they have been extracted from. For example, adrenal glandular is used to strengthen and stimulate weakened adrenal glands.

Glutathione—a protein composed of the amino acids cysteine, glutamic acid and glycine. It has antioxidant properties and assists the liver in detoxification.

Gluten—a protein component of certain grains that is found in wheat, oats, barley and rye.

Grape Seed Extract—contains PCOs (procyanidolic oligomers), a group of plant flavonoids known to have many beneficial health benefits. PCOs exert potent effects that protect body tissues and cells from oxidative damage. It is believed that PCOs have an antioxidant activity fifty times greater than vitamin C. Grape seed extract is commonly used for allergies, cardiovascular disease and prevention, immune enhancement, circulatory disorders, connective tissue disorders and as a general antioxidant.

Homeopathic physician—a physician who has specialized training in the use of homeopathy.

Homeopathy—system of medicine that uses minute doses of a substance to stimulate a healing response by the body's innate healing powers. Based on theory that "like cures like" whereby a substance that can cause symptoms in a healthy person can cure those same symptoms in an ill person.

Hypoallergenic—low potential for allergic reaction.

Hypoglycemia—low blood sugar.

Immune system—the body's defense system which protects against foreign substances or organisms.

Inflammation—the reaction of the body to tissue injury. Typical signs are redness, heat, swelling and pain.

IU—International Units, a unit of measurement for vitamins.

Kamut—a relative of durum wheat that may be tolerated better by people with a wheat sensitivity (not gluten allergy).

Laxative—a substance or food that promotes the movement of the bowels and prevents constipation.

Lecithin—a phospholipid mixture of fatty acids, glycerol, phosphorus, choline or inositol that is a normal part of the cell membrane.

L-Tryptophan—an essential amino acid that is necessary for proper growth and development. It is a precursor to the brain chemical serotonin which is involved in mood enhancement.

Lysine—an amino acid needed for growth and which has an inhibitory effect on the *herpes simplex* virus.

Malabsorption—defective absorption of nutrients by the intestines into the bloodstream. Improper absorption of foodstuffs can lead to build-up of disease-promoting toxins.

Massage—external pressure applied to the skin and muscles of the body. It is used for muscle and nerve relaxation, improved circulation and elimination of waste products.

Massage therapist—a therapist certified in the health care field of massage. There are various techniques of massage in which one can be trained.

Mental imagery—the use of visualization to relax or train the body. It is currently being used in the medical community for its benefits on the immune system function and other health related areas. For example, cancer patients can visualize the immune system killing cancer cells. It is widely used by athletes for training and preparation for competition.

Metabolism—a process of chemical and physical change for efficient utilization.

Methionine—an amino acid used by the body for growth and detoxification.

Mineral—an inorganic element or compound occurring naturally. The body cannot synthesize its own minerals. They are needed for the proper function of vitamins and other enzyme systems.

Mucous membranes—the inside lining of body cavities such as the respiratory and digestive tracts.

Neurotransmitter—a chemical nerve impulse used by the brain and nervous system for communication.

N-Acetylcysteine—an amino acid complex that is used to dissolve mucus and detoxify heavy metals from the body.

Naturopathic doctor—a physician trained in conventional and natural medicine in a four year medical school. They focus on the use of treatments that emphasize the body's inherent healing mechanisms.

Nutrient—a substance required by the body for growth and to maintain life.

Organic—used in this book in reference to foods grown without pesticides, herbicides, hormones or other chemicals.

Phenylalanine—an essential amino acid that is used by the body as a neurotransmitter. It is used clinically for mood enhancement and pain control.

Physiotherapy—the use of external therapies to prevent and treat health conditions. This includes the used of heat, cold, light and physical and mechanical means to enhance the body's healing powers. Physiotherapists are trained health care specialists in the use of physiotherapy.

Plant enzymes—purified enzymes derived from plant sources and which are commonly used to aid digestion.

Protein—a combination of amino acids required by the body for the formation of body tissues, enzymes, hormones and creation of energy.

Quercitin—a bioflavonoid used as a natural antihistamine.

Quinoa—a grain that contains more protein than any other. It is also relatively high in fiber, minerals, vitamins and the essential fatty acids. It is commonly used as an alternative for people with wheat sensitivity (not gluten allergy).

RDA—estimate by a U.S. government agency to establish nutritional needs for satisfactory growth of children and prevention of nutrient depletion in adults. There is much debate among nutrition-oriented physicians over the the low dosages recommended.

Rhizome—plant roots extending underneath or above the ground.

SAD—Seasonal Affective Disorder. Persons afflicted with this condition are prone to bouts of depression during the darker winter months. Symptoms are relieved with exposure to sunlight or ultraviolet rays.

Saturated fat—a fat with the maximum number of bonded

hydrogens and that is solid at room temperature. It is found in animal and dairy products.

Shark cartilage—refers to the powdered shark cartilage presently being used in the treatment of cancer. It appears to have immune stimulating properties, as well as the ability to cut off the blood supply to tumors thus shrinking them by starvation. It is also used in the treatment of arthritis and psoriasis.

Spelt—a relative of wheat often used by people with a wheat sensitivity, as it is easier to digest. It should not be used by people with gluten allergy.

Spinal manipulation—the use of joint mobilization to promote optimal nerve and circulation flow.

T'ai chi—a gentle form of Chinese martial arts that involves performing a slow, controlled sequence of movements. The goal is to harmonize the flow of energy (chi) through the body and promote a balance between mind and body.

Taurine—an amino acid that is involved in bile formation. It is also used for heart muscle conditions such as congestive heart failure and other specific conditions.

Toxin—a poison from environmental (food, water, air) or internal production (malabsorption in the digestive tract).

Triglyceride—a compound composed of three fatty acids and glycerol. It can be a fat in the blood or diet.

Tyrosine—an amino acid that is a precursor to neurotransmitters. It is used for conditions such as hypothyroidism and depression.

Unsaturated fat—a fat that is liquid at room temperature. It is a primary component of essential fatty acids such as flaxseed oil.

Vitamin—an organic substance required for the functioning of the body. Humans can synthesize a small number of vitamins, the rest must be acquired through the diet or supplementation.

Water soluble—able to dissolve in water. For example, vitamin C is water soluble so it does not need fat to be absorbed.

Resources

American Association of
Naturopathic Physicians
(AANP)
601 Valley Street, Suite #105
Seattle, WA 98109
(206) 298-0125
AANP website http://www.infi-
nite.org/Naturopathic.Physician

Bastyr University
14500 Juanito Drive NE
Bothell, WA 98011
(425) 823-1300

Canadian Association of
Naturopathic Physicians
4174 Dundas Street W,
Suite #304
Etobicoke, ON M8X 1X3
(416) 233-1043

The Canadian College of
Naturopathic Medicine
Box 2431, 2300 Yonge Street,
18th Floor
Toronto, ON M4P 1E4
(416) 486-8584

Homeopathic Academy of
Naturopathic Physicians
P.O. Box 69565
Portland, OR 97201
(503) 795-0579

International Foundation
for Homeopathy (IFH)
P.O. Box 7
Edmonds, WA 98020
(206) 776-1499

National College of
Naturopathic Medicine
049 SW Porter Street
Portland, OR 97201
(503) 499-4343

Natural Factors
3655 Bonneville Place
Burnaby, BC V3N 4S9
(604) 420-4229

Southwest College of
Naturopathic Medicine and
Health Sciences
2140 East Broadway Road
Tempe, AZ 85282
(602) 858-9100

University of Bridgeport,
College of Naturopathic
Medicine
221 University Avenue
Bridgeport, CT 06601
(203) 576-4109

References

I recommend the following references as educational resources for my readers.

American Association of Naturopathic Physicians. *Naturopathic Medicine: What it is...What it can do for you.* Seattle: AANP, 1991.

Boyle, W. and Saine, A. *Lectures in Naturopathic Hydrotherapy.* East Palestine: Buckeye Naturopathic Press, 1988.

Erasmus, Udo. *Fats that Heal. Fats that Kill.* Burnaby: Alive Books, 1993.

Gaby, A. *Preventing and Reversing Osteoporosis.* Rocklin: Prima Publishing, 1994.

Gladstar, R. *Herbal Healing for Women.* New York: Fireside Books, 1993.

Hudson, T. *Gynecology and Naturopathic Medicine.* Portland: TK Publications, 1992.

Lust, J. *The Herb Book.* New York: Bantam Books, 1974.

Mindell, E. *Vitamin Bible.* New York: Warner Books, Inc., 1991.

Morrison, R. *Desktop Guide.* Berkeley: Hahnemann Clinic Publishing, 1993.

Murray, M. *Encyclopedia of Nutritional Supplements.* Rocklin: Prima Publishing, 1996.

Reichenberg, J. and Ullman, R. *Ritalin Free Kids.* Rocklin: Prima Publishing, 1996.

Sahelian, R. and Tuttle, D. *Creatine Nature's Muscle Builder.* Garden City Park: Avery Publishing Company, 1977.

Thomas, C. *Taber's Cyclopedic Medical Dictionary.* Philadelphia: F.A. Davis Company, 1993.

Werbach, M. *Healing With Food.* Harper Perennial, 1993.

Weil, A. Natural Health, Natural Medicine. Boston: Houghton Mifflin Company, 1990.

Index

A

Absorption, 13-14, 19-20, 57, 98, 109, 173, 175, 178-194, 198, 203
Acetyl-L-Carnitine, 12, 198
Acidophilus, 40, 91, 95, 118, 128-129, 137
Acne, 9-11, 153, 163, 177, 182, 187, 189, 194
Aconite, 147
Acupressure, 5
Acupuncture, 3, 5, 13, 16, 19, 21, 28, 36, 39, 41, 43, 49, 64, 68, 70-71, 76, 79, 83, 85, 90, 92, 95, 98-99, 101, 103, 105, 107-108, 113-114, 116, 119, 122-125, 129, 132, 198, 209
Adaptogen, 156, 164, 198
ADHD, 85, 182
Adrenal glands, 64, 124, 162, 198, 200-201
Adrenal glandular, 64, 87, 105, 201
AIDS, 27, 76, 83-85, 122, 182, 184-185, 189, 194, 199
Alanine, 114
Allergens, 22, 117, 133, 136
Aloe, 34, 126, 156, 189
Aluminum, 12, 86
Alzheimer's, 11-13, 161, 182-183, 198
Amaranth, 61-62, 68, 109, 168, 171, 198
American ginseng, 26, 156
Amino acid, 47-48, 56, 180, 183, 191, 198, 202-205
Anemia, 13-14, 33, 101, 149, 153, 164-165, 176, 179, 182, 184, 187-188, 190-191, 194
Angelica, 10, 100, 102, 112, 157
Angina, 14-16, 161, 188
Antacid, 77
Anti-inflammatory, 18-19, 21, 26, 28, 35-36, 41, 44, 72, 74, 90, 94, 98-99, 102, 104-105, 114, 117, 121-122, 127, 131, 157-158, 162, 164, 198-199
Antioxidant, 12, 16, 38, 42-43, 45, 84, 99, 104, 117, 131, 177-178, 185, 188, 191-192, 194, 198, 201-202
Anxiety, 16-18, 92, 148-149, 153, 161-163
Apis, 29, 145, 147

Arginine, 47, 200

Arnica, 27, 29-30, 33, 121-122, 147-148, 157
Aromatherapy, 123
Arsenicum, 148
Arteriosclerosis, 88-89, 187
Artery, 11, 13, 15-16, 22-24, 26, 37, 59, 78-79, 84, 89, 105, 199-200
Arthritis, 18-20, 141, 145, 147-148, 151, 159, 170, 179, 181, 185-186, 188, 193-194, 199-200, 205, 210
Artificial sweeteners, 15, 55, 90, 93, 123, 134, 167
Asthma, 20-22, 141, 148, 150-151, 153, 160, 162, 182, 185, 190-191
Astragalus, 37, 46, 65, 84, 157
Astringent, 161, 199
Atherosclerosis, 15, 22-24, 57, 77-78, 162, 182, 184, 199
Athlete's foot, 24-25
Athletic performance enhancement, 25
Autoimmune condition, 199
Autoimmune disease, 98
Avena sativa, 17, 96, 162

B

B complex, 12, 16-17, 21, 23, 38, 40-41, 43, 54, 56, 58, 63, 66, 68, 72, 76, 79, 84, 87, 92, 94, 96-97, 102, 104, 106-107, 113, 116, 124-125, 127, 135
Bach flower remedy, 199
Bearberry, 157
Belladonna, 148
Berberis, 10, 97
Beta-carotene, 31-32, 38, 42-43, 45-46, 52, 61, 111, 117, 120, 132, 137, 173, 176-177, 198
Betaine HCl, 20-21, 91, 110, 116, 199
Bilberry, 42, 58, 130, 157
Bile, 70-72, 157-158, 164, 205
Biochemical imbalances, 17, 134
Biofeedback, 5, 83, 126, 199
Biofeedback training, 126
Bioflavonoid, 199, 204
Bioflavonoids, 14, 19, 21, 23, 25, 27-29, 31-35, 38, 40, 43, 45-46, 48, 51-54, 58,

61, 63, 65, 68, 71, 73-74, 79-80, 82, 84, 87, 96-97, 99, 111, 117, 119-120, 122, 124-125, 129, 131-132, 137, 185
Biomechanics, 42
Biotin, 54, 176, 182
Birth control pill, 45
Bites and stings, 28-29
Black currant, 54, 104, 157
Black currant oil, 54, 104
Black eye, 29-30
Blackstrap molasses, 13, 69, 108, 190
Blisters, 47
Blood sugar, 11, 17-18, 25, 27, 43, 57-59, 92, 105, 134-135, 162, 167, 181, 187, 194, 202
Blood vessels, 16, 23, 29, 32, 58, 79-80, 82, 106, 131, 139, 157, 185
Blue cohosh, 102, 157
Blue-green algae, 27, 33, 38, 199
Boils, 30-31, 148, 153, 177
Boric acid, 137
Boron, 69, 109, 173, 176, 186
Botanical medicine, 4-5, 154
Bovine cartilage, 39, 199
Breast-feeding, 48-49, 61
Brewer's yeast, 13, 47, 49, 58, 81, 179-181, 184-185, 187, 192
Bromelain, 16, 19, 23, 29, 33, 35, 41, 72, 79, 121, 131, 199
Bronchial tubes, 31-32, 51
Bronchitis, 31-32, 141, 148-151, 153, 159-160, 162, 170
Bruises, 29, 32-33, 148, 150, 157
Bryonia, 148
Burdock, 10, 24, 37, 54, 66, 75, 115, 117, 135, 157
Burns, 33-34, 133, 148, 156, 178, 185
Bursa, 34
Bursitis, 34-36, 149, 182
Butcher's broom, 80, 130, 157

C
Cactus, 15-16, 158
Cadmium, 83, 98
Caffeine, 9, 12, 15, 17-18, 22, 24, 26, 35-36, 41-42, 44, 49, 51, 55, 62, 68, 70, 72, 75, 78, 80, 84, 89-90, 92-93, 97-98, 100-101, 104-105, 108, 110, 112, 114-115, 121, 123, 126, 134, 136, 171
Calc fluor, 20, 43, 74, 81, 110, 122, 131, 152

Calc phos, 14, 20, 70, 106, 110, 153
Calc sulph, 153
Calcium, 17, 21-22, 27, 35, 41, 51, 68-70, 76-77, 82, 86, 92, 96-97, 100-102, 104-106, 108-110, 113, 125, 149, 152-153, 173, 176, 178, 186, 189-191, 195
Calendula, 11, 24, 28, 34, 53, 117, 137, 158
Cancer, 36-39, 44, 139, 141, 148, 163, 166, 178, 185, 188-191, 193, 199, 203, 205, 210
Canker sores, 39-40, 180, 184
Cantharis, 34, 129, 148
Carbohydrates, 25-26, 56-57, 92, 133-135, 179-180, 182, 199
Carbuncle, 30
Carpal tunnel syndrome, 40-42, 182
Cartilage, 38-39, 116, 191, 193, 199-200, 205
Cascara, 51, 158
Cat's claw, 19, 24, 127, 158
Cataracts, 42-43, 153, 157-158, 178, 180, 185
Causticum, 34
Cayenne, 23, 53, 106, 158
Cell, 27, 38, 86, 139, 152, 166, 179, 181-184, 198, 200-202
Cell salts, 152
Cervical dysplasia, 43-45, 177, 184-185
Chamomile, 17, 49, 62, 77, 91, 94, 117, 123, 125, 127, 149, 158
Chamomile tea, 49, 77, 91, 94, 123, 125
Charcoal capsules, 60, 200
Charcoal poultice, 29
Chasteberry, 158
Chelated minerals, 200
Chelation therapy, 13, 16, 23, 79, 83, 200
Cherry bark, 31, 52, 158
Child, 49, 60-61, 85-86, 156
Children, 13, 59-62, 65, 85-86, 105, 146, 149, 152, 174, 178, 188, 190, 204
Chimaphila, 129, 163
Chinese herbal medicine, 14, 19, 24, 32-33, 39, 43, 59, 64, 68, 71, 79, 81, 85, 95, 98-99, 101, 114, 116, 119, 128-129, 131-132, 137
Chionanthus, 158
Chiropractic, 28, 36, 41, 49, 62, 76, 125, 200
Chlorine, 26

Chlorophyll, 14, 38, 199-200
Cholesterol, 16, 22-23, 70-71, 78, 82, 88, 158, 161, 180-181, 183-185, 187, 200, 210
Choline, 71, 176, 183-184, 202
Chromium, 11, 18, 23, 25, 27, 58, 135, 173, 176, 180, 187
Cimicifuga, 157
Cineraria, 42, 158
Cinnamon, 65, 106, 159
Cinnamon tea, 65, 106
Clinical nutrition, 3-4
Cobalt, 187
Coenzyme Q10, 12, 16, 23, 27, 38, 63, 74, 79, 82, 84, 131, 188
Colchicum, 73
Cold, 4, 11, 15, 20, 22, 26, 30, 33, 37, 44-48, 57, 60, 62, 78, 84, 86, 89, 103, 111, 115, 118-119, 121-122, 139-140, 142-143, 147-153, 204
Cold-pressed oils, 11, 15, 22, 26, 37, 44, 78, 83, 88, 104, 166
Cold sores, 47-48, 153
Cold water fish, 11, 15, 20, 22, 26, 37, 44, 57, 78, 84, 89, 103, 115
Colic, 48-49, 149, 170
Collinsonia, 80, 159
Colon, 51, 94, 167, 178
Coltsfoot, 159
Comfrey, 53, 69, 152, 159, 189
Complex carbohydrates, 26, 57, 92, 133-134
Compress, 69, 117, 119, 121-122, 155
Conjunctivitis, 110-112, 151-152, 160
Connective tissue, 20, 27, 35, 121-123, 125, 157, 161, 185, 187-189, 191, 193, 200, 202
Constipation, 50-51, 80, 86, 93, 141, 151, 160, 170, 186, 190, 202
Constitutional hydrotherapy, 19, 28, 32, 39, 45-46, 49, 52, 60, 62, 65, 67-68, 71, 73, 79, 81, 85, 88, 91, 93, 95, 98-99, 103, 115-116, 118, 121, 128-129, 131, 141-142
Copper, 10, 12, 25, 31, 34, 38, 40, 43, 48, 53-54, 58, 69, 84, 87, 106, 109, 114, 116, 119, 122, 124, 127, 132, 137, 173, 176, 187, 191, 194
Cough, 32, 51-52, 148, 151, 158-159, 162
Counseling, 3, 5, 22, 39, 56, 83, 85-86, 90, 124, 127, 136
Cradle cap, 54, 183

Crampbark, 102, 112, 159
Cranberry, 82, 97, 128-129, 159
Craniosacral therapy, 126
Creatine, 27, 200, 207
Curcuma, 104, 164
Curcumin, 41, 122
Cuts, 53, 153, 158
Cynara, 161

D

Dairy alternatives, 10, 18, 24, 31, 35, 52, 61
Dandelion, 41, 44, 50, 66, 68, 71-72, 75, 82, 91, 94, 102, 107, 109, 113, 135, 159
Dandruff, 53-55
Decoction, 154-155
Depression, 55-57, 86, 148, 150, 153, 157, 161, 164, 170, 179-180, 182-185, 188-189, 194, 204-205
Detox Juicing Recipe, 135
Detoxification, 10, 26, 71, 117, 134, 140, 162, 166, 180-181, 188, 191, 201, 203
Devil's claw, 35, 72, 159, 210
DHEA, 13, 20-21, 56, 59, 63, 88, 90, 99, 101, 105, 110, 198, 200
Diabetes, 43, 57-59, 133, 161, 178, 180, 182-185, 187-188, 190-191, 194
Diarrhea, 38, 59-60, 84, 93, 110, 141, 148-149, 160, 163, 170, 180-181, 185, 188, 191-194
Diathermy, 4
Digestive tract, 49, 59-60, 93-94, 127-128, 140, 152, 156, 158, 205
Dioscorea, 71, 75, 100, 164
Diuretic, 82, 159, 161, 200
DNA, 45, 200
Dong quai, 10, 100, 102, 112, 157

E

Ear infections, 60-62, 148, 170
Echinacea, 30, 32, 37, 46, 52, 61, 64, 84, 111, 118, 120, 129, 132, 136, 159
Electrical pulses, 4
Electrolytes, 25, 59
Elimination and reintroduction diet, 55, 67, 70, 90, 107, 117, 136, 170
Enzyme, 167, 173, 188, 191, 199-200, 203
Ephedra, 21, 119, 160

Equisetum, 161
Essential fatty acids, 10-11, 15-16, 19-20, 22-23, 26, 35, 37-38, 44, 54, 57, 66, 78, 82, 84-85, 89, 94, 99-100, 102, 104, 113-117, 135, 201, 204-205
Estrogen, 100, 110, 112-113, 136, 186, 201
Euphrasia, 111, 160
Evening primrose, 66, 100, 102, 113, 160
Evening primrose oil, 66, 100, 102, 113
Exercise, 3-4, 11, 16, 18, 20, 24, 39, 51, 56, 59, 64, 76-77, 79-80, 83, 85, 88, 90, 93, 95, 105, 108, 110, 113, 115, 124, 127, 131, 133, 135
Exercise therapy, 3-4
Eyebright, 43, 111, 160
Eyewash, 111

F
Fast, 20, 25, 30, 35, 68, 73, 90, 93, 174
Fat, 9, 11, 15, 22, 36, 44, 70, 78, 83, 88, 97, 100, 103, 133-135, 162, 166, 173, 177-179, 182-184, 191, 200-201, 204-205
Fat soluble, 173, 177-179, 200-201
Fat soluble vitamins, 173, 177
Fatigue, 13, 45, 55, 62-64, 100, 128, 141, 149, 151, 153, 156, 164, 170, 179-182, 184, 188-191, 193
Fatty acids, 10-11, 13, 15-16, 19-20, 22-24, 26-27, 35-38, 44, 54-55, 57, 59, 66, 78-79, 82, 84-85, 89, 94, 99-100, 102, 104-105, 113-118, 133, 135, 166, 180, 201-202, 204-205
Fennel, 49, 160
Fennel tea, 49
Fenugreek, 58
Ferrum phos, 14, 33, 36, 65, 149, 153
Fever, 30-31, 45-47, 60, 64-65, 118, 128, 139-140, 147-149, 153
Feverfew, 76, 160
Fiber, 10-11, 15, 22, 26, 36, 44, 50, 57, 66, 70, 78, 80-81, 83, 88, 93-94, 97, 100, 112, 115, 126, 130, 133-134, 167, 204
Fibrocystic breast disease, 65-67, 170, 178
Flax, 160
Flaxseed oil, 10-11, 15-16, 19, 22-23, 26, 35, 37-38, 44, 50, 54, 66, 78, 82-83, 85,

89, 94, 99-100, 102, 104, 114, 116-117, 132, 135, 167, 169, 205
Fluoride, 152, 188
Folic acid, 12-14, 45, 64, 69, 73-74, 104, 109, 176, 182-185
Food allergies and sensitivities, 9, 20, 30, 39, 47, 50, 52, 55, 57, 59, 61, 63, 67, 80, 82, 98, 103, 112, 115, 118, 126, 128, 133, 135, 170, 172
Food allergy, 201
Food sensitivity, 107, 201
Foot hydrotherapy, 47, 62, 65, 76, 92, 107, 112, 119, 121, 131, 139, 141-142
Fractures, 68-70, 108, 152-153, 178
Free radical, 42, 131, 198, 201
Fructo-oligosaccharides, 95
Fungal infection, 24

G
Gall-bladder, 68, 70-72, 91, 94, 135, 158, 161, 170
Gallstones, 70-71
Garcinia, 160
Garlic capsules, 32, 46, 52
Garlic, 12, 15-16, 22-24, 26, 32, 37, 44, 46, 52, 58, 61, 78, 81-82, 84, 89, 120, 130, 132, 136, 160, 189
Garlic oil drops, 61
Gelsemium, 96, 149
Gentian root, 10, 14, 21, 50, 67, 75, 91, 94, 98, 109, 117, 160
Geranium, 127, 160
Germanium, 173, 189
Ginger root, 19, 50, 65, 68, 75, 91, 94, 154, 160
Gingivitis, 73-74, 184, 188
Ginkgo, 12, 15, 23, 26, 42, 79, 82, 86, 89, 104, 106, 161
Ginseng, 12, 26, 63, 89, 95, 123, 156, 164, 189
Glands, 9, 26-27, 53, 59, 63-64, 79, 87, 95, 98-99, 101, 105, 123-124, 156, 162-163, 181, 198, 200-201
Glandular connective tissue complex, 123
Glandular extracts, 20
Glandular, 14, 20, 39, 56, 59, 63-64, 87-89, 101, 105, 123, 136, 201
Glandular treatment, 59, 101
Globe artichoke, 161

Glucosamine sulfate, 19, 36, 122
Glutamic acid, 114, 201
Glutamine, 127
Gluten, 201-202, 204-205
Glycine, 114, 200-201
Goldenseal, 30-31, 39, 44, 46, 52, 59, 64,
    73, 111, 118, 120, 129, 136, 161
Gotu kola, 55, 85, 161
Gout, 71-73, 184-185, 191
Grape seed extract, 19, 27, 35, 38, 43,
    74, 79-80, 86, 99, 104, 119, 131, 201-
    202
Gugulipid, 23, 161
Gum Disease, 73-74
Gymnemma, 58, 161

H

Hammamelis, 131, 164
Hawthorn berry, 82, 130
Hawthorn, 15, 78, 82, 130, 161
HCA, 135, 160
Headache, 45, 74-76, 112, 148-150, 171,
    177, 180, 191
Heart attack, 22
Heart disease, 77-79, 133, 161, 166-167,
    178-179, 188, 190, 193
Heart, 1, 14-16, 22, 77-79, 82, 98, 133,
    158, 161, 166-167, 178-179, 183, 186-
    188, 190-193, 199, 205
Heartburn, 76-77, 141, 153
Hemoglobin, 13
Hemorrhoids, 79-81, 141, 153, 157, 159,
    161, 164, 170
Hepar sulph, 31, 149
Herbal medicine, 3, 14, 19, 24, 32-33, 39,
    43, 59, 64, 68, 71, 79, 81, 85, 95, 98-99,
    101, 114, 116, 119, 128-129, 131-132,
    137, 154
Herpes, 47-48, 147-148, 151, 179, 202
High blood pressure, 15, 22, 24, 77, 81-
    83, 90, 159, 161, 167, 180, 191-193
HIV, 83-85, 163
Homeopathic physician, 4, 202
Homeopathic Rescue Remedy, 18, 90,
    96, 124
Homeopathy, 3-4, 9, 12, 19, 21, 32, 39,
    45, 49, 56, 58, 62, 68, 73, 76, 85-87, 90,
    95, 99, 101, 103, 105, 113, 115-116,
    119, 128-129, 132, 137, 144-146, 152,
    202, 206

Hormonal imbalance, 9, 65, 88, 101,
    136, 163
Hormone imbalance, 66, 75, 98, 163-164
Hormone replacement therapy, 100
Horse chestnut, 80, 130, 161
Horseradish, 118, 161
Horsetail, 129, 161, 193
Hydrochloric acid, 21, 199
Hydrotherapy, 3-4, 9, 19, 28, 32, 39, 45-
    47, 49, 52, 60, 62, 65, 67-68, 71, 73, 76,
    79, 81, 85, 88, 91-93, 95, 98-99, 103,
    107, 112, 115-116, 118-119, 121, 123,
    128-129, 131, 139-142, 207
    see also Constitutional Hydrother-
    apy
    see also Foot Hydrotherapy
Hyperactivity, 85-86
Hypericum, 84, 149, 164
Hypertension, 81-82, 88, 141, 185-186,
    188, 190, 192
Hypnosis, 22, 48, 132, 135
Hypoallergenic, 202
Hypoglycemia, 17, 187, 191, 202
Hypothyroid, 86-88
Hypothyroidism, 55, 162, 177, 189, 205

I

IBS, 93-94
Ignatia, 149
Immune system, 25, 27, 31, 37-39, 44,
    46-48, 52, 59, 61, 64-65, 67, 83-85, 96,
    98-99, 103, 111, 118-120, 129, 131-
    132, 136-137, 139-141, 144, 158, 163,
    167, 170, 177, 188, 190, 194, 199, 201-
    203
Impotence, 88-90, 141
Indigestion, 90-91
Infant, 48-49, 54
Infection, 24, 28, 30-31, 51, 53, 59-60, 96,
    98, 110, 118, 120, 128, 136-137, 141,
    145, 147-151, 153, 157, 159, 161-163
Inflammation, 18-20, 35-36, 41, 59, 68,
    71-74, 99, 102, 110, 114-116, 120-121,
    126-127, 131, 151, 153, 181-182, 187,
    198, 202
Infusion, 154-155
Inositol, 23, 176, 181, 183-184, 202
Insomnia, 91-93, 142, 163-164, 201
Iodine, 10, 87, 173, 176, 189
Ipecac, 107, 150

Iron deficiency, 14, 176, 190
Iron, 12-14, 19, 23, 25, 27, 32, 34, 38, 40, 43, 45-46, 54, 63-64, 74, 91, 94, 99, 101, 104, 106, 110, 116, 119, 122, 124, 135, 137, 149, 173, 176, 185, 190
Irritable bowel syndrome, 93-95, 141, 170

J
Jet lag, 95-96
Juice fast, 20, 25, 30, 35, 68, 73

K
Kali bich, 150
Kali mur, 153
Kali sulph, 153
Kamut, 202
Kava kava, 17, 56, 125, 161
Kelp, 87, 162, 179, 186, 189
Kidney stones, 96-98, 157, 182, 191

L
L-Carnitine, 16, 27, 79, 135
L-Glutamine, 94
L-Glutathione, 117
L-Tryptophan, 56, 202
Lactic acid, 28
Laxative, 50-51, 156, 158, 202
Lecithin, 12, 23, 71, 179, 184, 202
Ledum, 29, 150
Licorice, 18, 21, 26, 37, 40, 44, 47, 77, 98, 100, 104, 112, 127, 162
Liniment, 155
Liver glandular extract, 14
Liver, 10, 13-14, 26, 37, 44, 63, 66, 68, 70-72, 75, 91, 94, 99, 102-103, 107, 112, 115-116, 135, 140, 157-159, 161-162, 173, 177-181, 183-185, 187-188, 190, 192, 195, 201
Lomatium, 47, 132, 162
Lupus, 98-99, 141, 178, 200
Lycopodium, 150
Lysine, 47-48, 202

M
Mag phos, 42, 86, 91, 103, 105-106, 126, 153
Magnesium, 16-17, 21, 27, 35, 41, 51, 58, 60, 63, 70, 76, 79, 82, 86, 92, 97, 101-102, 104-106, 110, 113, 125, 131, 135, 153, 173, 175, 176, 182, 186, 190-191
Malabsorption, 93, 203, 205
Manganese, 69, 109, 122, 173, 176, 191
Marshmallow, 32, 60, 120, 129, 162
Massage, 28, 42, 49, 76, 123, 125, 155, 203
Massage therapist, 203
Melatonin, 56, 92, 96
Menopause, 99-101, 157-158, 186, 210
Menstrual cramps, 101-103, 141, 151, 157, 163
Mental imagery, 16, 18, 22, 28, 39, 79, 83, 85, 93, 95, 105, 124, 127, 203
Mercury, 74, 145, 151, 210
Metabolism, 12, 59, 71-72, 86, 88, 97, 99, 133-136, 166, 173, 178-180, 182-184, 191, 203
Methionine, 200, 203
Milk thistle, 10, 26, 37, 63, 66, 71, 75, 99, 113, 116, 162, 195
Mineral, 9, 13-14, 42, 73, 106, 124, 135, 144, 173-176, 186, 197, 203
Molybdenum, 173, 176, 191
MSG, 75, 167, 171
Mucus, 31, 51-52, 93, 118-119, 203
Mullein, 21, 52, 61, 162
Multi-vitamin, 12, 14, 19, 21, 23, 25, 27, 33-34, 38, 40, 43, 45-46, 54, 58, 60, 63, 74, 84, 86, 91, 94, 96, 99, 101, 104, 106, 110, 116, 119, 122, 124, 135, 137, 175-176
Multiple sclerosis, 103-105, 141, 149, 160, 179, 182
Muscle cramps, 105, 153, 180, 186, 190
Muscle, 16, 19, 25, 27, 76, 79, 93, 102-103, 105-107, 122, 124, 126, 135, 149, 151, 153, 157, 161, 180, 182-183, 186-187, 190-193, 199, 203, 205, 207
Myrrh, 39, 73, 162

N
N-Acetylcysteine, 119, 203
Nat mur, 48, 153
Nat phos, 28, 40, 73, 77, 128, 153
Nat sulph, 153
Natural childbirth, 3-4
Natural vitamins, 174
Naturopathic doctor, 203
Nausea, 28, 46, 70, 75, 107-108, 150, 163, 179, 182, 185, 188, 192-194

Nerve, 13, 16, 27, 40-41, 57, 59, 103-105, 123, 149, 153, 162, 179, 181-182, 184, 186-187, 190, 192-193, 200, 203, 205
Nervous system, 12, 17-18, 48, 51, 56, 63-64, 76, 85-86, 96, 99, 102-103, 105, 123-125, 141, 151, 167, 179, 182-183, 188, 191, 199-200, 203
Neurotransmitter, 12, 56, 183, 186, 188, 198, 203-204
Nutrient, 16, 79, 122, 174, 200, 204, 210
Nutritional balancing, 5
Nux vomica, 91, 107, 128, 151

O

Oatmeal bath, 118
Oatmeal, 11, 118, 123, 168, 193
Oatstraw, 63, 123, 162
Obesity, 133
Oil, 9-11, 13, 15-16, 19, 22-24, 26-27, 29, 35-38, 44, 49-50, 53-55, 59, 61, 66, 78-79, 82-85, 88-89, 94, 99-100, 102-105, 113-119, 121, 132-133, 135, 155, 157, 162, 167, 169, 177-179, 187, 205
Olive oil, 11, 15, 22, 26, 37, 44, 49, 54, 78, 83, 88-89, 104, 155, 167, 169
Onion, 32, 37, 162, 189
Orchic glandular, 89
Oregon grape, 162
Organic calf liver, 13
Organic, 13, 20, 37, 42, 87, 112, 166, 171, 173, 179, 196-197, 204-205, 210
Oriental botanical medicine, 5
Oriental medicine, 5, 209
Osteoarthritis, 18, 170, 180
Osteoporosis, 100, 108-110, 153, 178-179, 182, 184, 186, 188, 190-191, 193, 207
Oxalate, 96-97

P

PABA, 184
Panax ginseng, 26, 63
Panic attacks, 17
Pap smear, 43
Passion flower, 17, 85, 89, 92, 124, 163
Peppermint, 40, 49, 77, 90, 94, 127, 163
Peppermint tea, 40, 49, 77, 90, 94
Periodontal disease, 73
PCO, 19, 27, 35, 38, 43, 74, 79-80, 86, 99, 104, 119, 131, 201-202

pH, 97, 136
Phenylalanine, 204
Phosphorus, 151, 173, 178, 191-192, 202
Physical medicine, 3-4, 209
Physiotherapy, 4, 36, 42, 122, 204
Phytolacca, 66, 163
Pink eye, 110-112
Pipsissewa, 163
Pituitary glandular, 87
Plant enzymes, 67, 72, 75, 91, 94, 99, 116, 135, 204
PMS, 112-113, 141, 157-160, 182, 191
Pneumonia, 31, 141, 148, 151
Pollutants, 22, 32, 174
Potassium, 81-82, 105, 150, 153, 167, 173, 177, 192
Poultice, 29-30, 155
Precursors, 14, 100
Pregnancy, 41, 45, 79, 107, 186, 191
Pregnenolone, 21, 99, 105
Premenstrual Syndrome, 112
Preservatives, 15, 20, 75, 85-86, 90, 93, 167, 171
Progesterone, 67, 100-102, 110, 113, 136
Prostate enlargement, 113-115, 141
Protein, 25-26, 33, 58, 67-68, 71-72, 97, 109, 133-134, 166, 169, 181-182, 190, 198, 201, 204
Psoriasis, 115-116, 141, 153, 157, 178, 205
Psyllium, 10, 22, 36, 50, 57, 66, 70, 78, 80-81, 93, 112, 115, 126, 130, 134, 167
Pulsatilla, 111, 119, 151
Pumpkin seeds, 89, 114, 187, 194
Purine, 72
Pygeum africanum, 114

Q

Quercitin, 21, 68, 111, 127, 204
Quinoa, 61-62, 68, 109, 168, 171, 204

R

Rash, 98, 116-118, 183, 189, 193-194
Raspberry, 102, 163
RDA, 175, 177-194, 204
Recommended daily allowance, 175
Red blood cells, 13-14, 178, 182, 184, 190
Red clover, 37, 44, 163

Reishi mushroom, 37, 84, 163
Respiratory system, 20, 45
Respiratory tract, 21, 31-32, 46, 60, 120-121, 177
Rhizome, 160-161, 163-164, 204
Rhus tox, 27, 48, 122, 151
RICE, 122, 10, 18, 20, 24, 31, 35, 52, 61, 63, 68, 78, 88, 97, 109, 122, 126, 168-169, 171, 179, 181, 183-185, 193
Rice milk, 10, 18, 24, 31-32, 52, 61, 63, 126, 168-169, 171
Rose hip tea, 97
Rumex, 13, 165
Ruta, 41

S

SAD, 204
Sarsaparilla, 116, 163
Saturated fat, 11, 15, 22, 36, 44, 78, 83, 88, 103, 133, 166, 204
Saunas, 123
Saw palmetto, 89, 114, 163
Scutellaria, 163
Seasonal Affective Disorder, 55-56, 204
Second hand smoke, 62
Selenium, 11, 38, 43, 45, 48, 58, 104, 116-117, 173, 177, 192, 198
Senna, 51
Shark cartilage, 38-39, 116, 205
Shiitake mushroom, 37, 163, 189
Shock, 28, 147-148, 181, 190, 200
Siberian ginseng, 12, 26, 63, 89, 95, 123, 164
Silica, 153, 177, 210
Silicea, 31, 123, 153
Silicon, 12, 69, 109, 173, 193
Sinusitis, 118-119, 142, 150-151, 161, 170
Sitz baths, 81
Slippery elm, 59, 77, 120, 127, 164
Sodium, 15, 78, 81, 105, 153, 167, 173, 193
Sore throat, 119-121, 141, 147, 149, 153, 162, 164
Soy products, 26, 37, 100, 171
Soy, 10, 18, 24, 26, 31, 35, 37, 49, 52, 63, 68, 97, 100, 109, 126, 166, 168-169, 171, 179, 181
Spelt, 61-62, 68, 109, 171, 205
Spinal manipulation, 28, 36, 41, 62, 76, 125, 205

Sprains and strains, 121
St. John's wort, 17, 55, 84, 124, 149, 164, 196
Stinging nettle, 14, 106, 111, 164
Strep throat, 120
Stress management, 5
Stress, 5, 12, 15-18, 22, 26-27, 36, 38-40, 47, 63, 73-74, 76-77, 79, 83-85, 87-91, 93-96, 98-99, 105, 113, 123-127, 149, 156, 162, 164, 168, 174-175, 181, 198
Stroke, 22
Sulphur, 152
Sunlight, 116, 178, 204
Swank diet, 103
Symphytum, 70, 152, 159
Synthetic vitamins, 174

T

T'ai chi, 18, 39, 57, 64, 79, 85, 105, 124, 205
Taurine, 58, 71, 205
Tea, 13, 17-18, 24, 35, 38, 40-41, 46, 49, 59, 65-66, 72, 77, 90-92, 94, 97, 101-102, 106-107, 114, 117, 120, 123, 125, 127, 150, 154, 164, 168-169, 179, 188, 191, 210
Tea tree oil, 24
Tea tree, 24, 164
Testosterone, 88-90, 101, 136
Thuja oil, 132
Thuja, 132, 164
Thymus glandular, 39
Thyroid gland, 86-88, 136, 189
Thyroid glandular, 56, 63, 88, 136
Thyroid, 56, 59, 63, 86-88, 101, 134, 136, 187, 189, 192-193
Tincture, 14, 24, 33-34, 53, 111, 117, 130, 154-156
Tissue, 16, 18-20, 25, 27-30, 33-36, 39-41, 43, 53, 68, 71, 73-74, 80-81, 94, 104, 121-123, 125-126, 136, 139, 151-152, 157, 161-162, 164, 185, 187-189, 191, 193, 199-202
TMJ syndrome, 124-126
Toxin, 205
Trace minerals, 27, 58, 173
Triglyceride, 23, 161, 205
Tumeric, 71, 164
Tussilago, 52, 159
Tyrosine, 56, 205

U

Ulcers, 39, 126-128, 153, 158, 160-162, 177
Ultrasound, 4
Unsaturated fat, 205
Uric acid, 71-73, 96, 181
Urinary tract infection, 128, 145, 148, 150
Urtica urens, 72

V

Vaccinium myrtillus, 157
Vaginitis, 136, 153, 164, 170
Valerian, 17, 76, 92, 102, 123, 125, 164
Vanadium, 173, 177, 194
Varicose veins, 130-131, 141, 153, 157, 161
Vitamin A, 10, 34, 43, 45, 87, 111, 121, 127, 132, 173, 176-177, 194
Vitamin B, *see B complex*
Vitamin B1, 176, 179, 187
Vitamin B12, 12, 21, 35, 54, 56, 63-64, 99, 104, 176, 182, 184, 187
Vitamin B2, 176, 180
Vitamin B3, 180
Vitamin B5, 181
Vitamin B6, 41, 69, 86, 92, 97, 107, 109, 113, 175-176, 181
Vitamin C, 14, 19, 21, 23, 25, 27-29, 31-35, 38, 40, 43, 45-46, 48, 51-54, 58, 60-61, 63, 65, 68-69, 71, 73-74, 79-80, 82, 84, 87, 96-97, 99, 109, 111, 117, 119-120, 122, 124-125, 129, 131-132, 137, 173, 175-176, 185, 190, 199, 202, 205
Vitamin D, 69, 109, 173, 176, 178
Vitamin E, 10, 16, 19, 23, 33-35, 38, 43, 48, 53, 58, 66, 74, 80, 99, 101-102, 104-106, 113-114, 117, 122, 127, 131-132, 174, 176, 178
Vitamin K, 69, 109, 173, 176, 179
Vitamin, 9-10, 12, 14, 16, 19, 21, 23, 25, 27-29, 31-35, 38, 40-41, 43, 45-46, 48, 51-54, 56, 58, 60-61, 63-66, 68-69, 71, 73-74, 79-80, 82, 84, 86-87, 92, 96-97, 99, 101-102, 104-107, 109, 111, 113-114, 116-117, 119-122, 124-125, 127, 129, 131-132, 137, 173-182, 184-185, 187, 190, 194, 197-199, 202, 205, 207
Vitamins, 9-10, 12-14, 16-17, 19, 21, 23, 25, 27-29, 31-35, 38, 40-43, 45-46, 48-49, 51-54, 56, 58, 60-61, 63, 65-66, 68-69, 71-72, 74, 76-77, 79-80, 82, 84, 86-87, 89, 91-92, 94, 96-97, 99, 101-102, 104, 106-107, 109, 111, 113-114, 116-117, 119-120, 122, 124-125, 127, 129, 131-132, 135, 137, 166-167, 173-177, 179-185, 190, 196, 198-199, 201-205, 210
Vitex, 75, 100, 112, 158

W

Warts, 131-133, 150, 153, 164
Water soluble vitamins, 173, 179
Water soluble, 78, 88, 173, 179-185, 205
Weight loss, 71, 73, 133-136, 160, 170, 187
Wheat alternatives, 61
Wild yam, 100, 102, 164
Witch hazel tincture, 130
Witch hazel, 130, 164

Y

Yam, 100, 102, 164
Yarrow, 46, 65, 164
Yeast Infection, 136-137
Yellow dock, 165
Yoga, 18, 39, 79, 85, 105, 124
Yogurt, 39, 69, 106, 108, 136-137, 171
Yohimbe, 89, 165
Yucca, 19

Z

Zinc, 10, 12, 25, 31-32, 34, 38, 40, 43, 46, 48, 52-54, 58, 61, 69, 84, 87, 89, 97, 105-106, 109, 114, 116, 119-120, 122, 124, 127, 132, 137, 173, 177, 187-188, 194

About the Author

Dr. Mark Stengler is a family naturopathic physician, lecturer and author. He specializes in the enhancement of health using natural medicine. He received his medical training at the National College of Naturopathic Medicine in Portland, Oregon, where he was awarded the Doctorate of Naturopathic Medicine (ND) and Certification of Homeotherapeutics (CHT). In addition to a busy practice and work as a consultant to the health food industry, Dr. Stengler is completing his Master's degree in Acupuncture and Oriental Medicine (M.Ac.O.M.). He is an expert in the fields of nutritional, botanical, homeopathic and physical medicine. He is a member of the following organizations:

- American Association of Naturopathic Physicians
- Oregon Association of Naturopathic Physicians
- Canadian Association of Naturopathic Physicians
- Alberta Association of Naturopathic Physicians
- Homeopathic Academy of Naturopathic Physicians
- Oregon Acupuncture Association

Dr. Stengler provides family health care for all ages, from pediatrics to geriatrics. He is known for his innovation in developing treatment programs for chronic degenerative illnesses. Having studied with many of the premier holistic and conventional physicians, Dr. Stengler focuses on integrating natural and orthodox medicine in both his treatments and research.

Dr. Stengler practices at The Natural Physician Center in Beaverton, Oregon. Contact him at 503-526-8600 or e-mail: thenaturalphysician@usa.net or NaturalRx@aol.com

Other Titles by Alive

The All-in-One Guide to Herbs, Vitamins & Minerals
The quick and easy reference for everything you need to know.
Victoria Hogan, 64 pp softcover

Allergies: Disease in Disguise
How to heal your allergic condition permanently and naturally.
Carolee Bateson-Koch, DC, ND, 224 pp softcover

The Breuss Cancer Cure
Advice for prevention and natural treatment of cancer, leukemia and other seemingly incurable diseases.
Rudolf Breuss (translated from German), 112 pp softcover

Devil's Claw Root and Other Natural Remedies for Arthritis
A herbal remedy that has freed arthritis sufferers from crippling pain.
Rachel Carston (revised by Klaus Kaufmann), 128 pp softcover

Diet for All Reasons
Nutrition guide and recipe collection.
Paulette Eisen, 176 pp softcover

Eliminating Poison in Your Mouth
Overcoming mercury amalgam toxicity.
Klaus Kaufmann, 44 pp softcover

Fats That Heal. Fats That Kill.
The complete guide to fats, oils, cholesterol and human health.
Udo Erasmus, 480 pp softcover

For the Love of Food
The complete natural foods cookbook.
J.M. Martin, 484 pp hardcover

Healing with Herbal Juices
A practical guide to herbal juice therapy: nature's preventative medicine.
Siegfried Gursche, 256 pp softcover

Kefir Rediscovered!
The nutritional benefits of an ancient healing food.
Klaus Kaufmann, 100 pp softcover

Kombucha Rediscovered!
A guide to the medicinal benefits of an ancient healing tea.
Klaus Kaufmann, 96 pp softcover

Living with Green Power
Gourmet recipes for raw food.
Elysa Markowitz, 176 pp hardcover

Menopause Time for a Change
The menopause handbook for safe and effective natural self-care approaches.
Merri Lu Park, 304 pp softcover

Return to the Joy of Health
Natural medicine and alternative treatments for all your health complaints.
Dr. Zoltan Rona, 408 pp softcover

Silica—The Forgotten Nutrient
A guide to the vital role of organic vegetal silica in nutrition, health, longevity and medicine.
Klaus Kaufmann, 128 pp softcover

Silica—The Amazing Gel
For beautiful hair, skin and nails.
Klaus Kaufmann, 208 pp softcover

All books available at your local natural food store, or at
alive Books
7436 Fraser Park Drive, Burnaby
BC V5J 5B9 Canada
1-800-661-0303